Coping with Kidney Disease

Dr Tom Smith has been writing full time since 1977, after spending six years in general practice and seven years in medical research. He writes the 'Doctor, Doctor' column in the *Guardian* on Saturdays, and also has columns in the *Bradford Telegraph and Argus*, the *Lancashire Telegraph*, the *Carrick Gazette* and the *Galloway Gazette*. He has written two humorous books, *Doctor, Have You Got a Minute?* and *A Seaside Practice*, both published by Short Books. His other books for Sheldon Press include *Heart Attacks: Prevent and Survive*, *Living with Alzheimer's Disease*, *Coping Successfully with Prostate Cancer*, *Overcoming Back Pain*, *Coping with Bowel Cancer*, *Coping with Heartburn and Reflux*, *Coping with Age-Related Memory Loss*, *Skin Cancer: Prevent and Survive* and *How to Get the Best from Your Doctor*.

D0266923

Overcoming Common Problems Series

Selected titles

A full list of titles is available from Sheldon Press,
36 Causton Street, London SW1P 4ST and on our website at
www.sheldonpress.co.uk

Body Language: What You Need to Know
David Cohen

The Chronic Pain Diet Book
Neville Shone

The Complete Carer's Guide
Bridget McCall

The Confidence Book
Gordon Lamont

Coping Successfully with Varicose Veins
Christine Craggs-Hinton

Coping with Age-related Memory Loss
Dr Tom Smith

Coping with Compulsive Eating
Ruth Searle

Coping with Diabetes in Childhood and Adolescence
Dr Philippa Kaye

Coping with Diverticulitis
Peter Cartwright

Coping with Family Stress
Dr Peter Cheevers

Coping with Hay Fever
Christine Craggs-Hinton

Coping with Hearing Loss
Christine Craggs-Hinton

Coping with Kidney Disease
Dr Tom Smith

Coping with Polycystic Ovary Syndrome
Christine Craggs-Hinton

Coping with Radiotherapy
Dr Terry Priestman

Coping with Tinnitus
Christine Craggs-Hinton

Depression: Healing Emotional Distress
Linda Hurcombe

Every Woman's Guide to Digestive Health
Jill Eckersley

The Fertility Handbook
Dr Philippa Kaye

Free Yourself from Depression
Colin and Margaret Sutherland

Helping Children Cope with Grief
Rosemary Wells

How to Be a Healthy Weight
Philippa Pigache

How to Get the Best from Your Doctor
Dr Tom Smith

The IBS Healing Plan
Theresa Cheung

Living with Birthmarks and Blemishes
Gordon Lamont

Living with Eczema
Jill Eckersley

Living with Schizophrenia
Dr Neel Burton and Dr Phil Davison

Living with a Seriously Ill Child
Dr Jan Aldridge

The Multiple Sclerosis Diet Book
Tessa Buckley

Overcoming Anorexia
Professor J. Hubert Lacey, Christine Craggs-Hinton and Kate Robinson

Overcoming Emotional Abuse
Susan Elliot-Wright

Overcoming Hurt
Dr Windy Dryden

Overcoming Insomnia
Susan Elliot-Wright

Overcoming Shyness and Social Anxiety
Ruth Searle

Reducing Your Risk of Cancer
Dr Terry Priestman

Stammering: Advice for all ages
Renée Byrne and Louise Wright

Stress-related Illness
Dr Tim Cantopher

Tranquillizers and Antidepressants: When to start them, how to stop
Professor Malcolm Lader

The Traveller's Good Health Guide
Dr Ted Lankester

Treating Arthritis – More Drug-Free Ways
Margaret Hills

Overcoming Common Problems

Coping with Kidney Disease

DR TOM SMITH

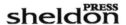

First published in Great Britain in 2008

Sheldon Press
36 Causton Street
London SW1P 4ST

The author and publisher have made every effort to ensure that the
external website and email addresses included in this book are correct and
up to date at the time of going to press. The author and publisher are not
responsible for the content, quality or continuing accessibility of the sites.

British Library Cataloguing-in-Publication Data
A catalogue record for this book is available from the British Library

ISBN 978-1-84709-036-2

1 3 5 7 9 10 8 6 4 2

Typeset by Fakenham Photosetting Ltd, Fakenham, Norfolk
Printed in Great Britain by Ashford Colour Press

Produced on paper from sustainable forests

For
Dr Mark MacGregor and his team
at Crosshouse Renal Unit,
Kilmarnock, Scotland

Contents

Note to the reader

This is not a medical book and is not intended to replace advice from your doctor. Consult your pharmacist or doctor if you believe you have any of the symptoms described, and if you think you might need medical help.

Introduction

James, at 62, feels well. He has never smoked, drinks only the odd glass of wine at the weekends, keeps fit by running regularly, and, being five feet nine tall and weighing just 12 stone, is in good shape. He has a healthy appetite, only feels tired at the appropriate time (that is, bedtime), sleeps well at night and is never wakened by the pressing need to go to the toilet. He considers himself fit, and so do all his family.

Naturally, when his doctor sent him a routine letter for a well-man check, he knew he would take it in his stride. He thought it would be 'a doddle'.

He was thunderstruck when one of his blood tests defined him as being in moderate chronic renal failure. How could this be? He had no symptoms, as far as he knew he had never had a kidney complaint, and he certainly did not feel in any way ill. Now it seemed that he was facing a long-term illness, with perhaps kidney dialysis and even transplant ahead of him.

His doctor was quick to reassure him. A fast calculation showed that James had less than a 1 per cent chance of his kidneys deteriorating so fast that he would eventually need dialysis. But he needed a few more tests, and he would have to return regularly, perhaps every 3 months to begin with, for further checks on his kidney function, just to make sure.

I have written this book for the hundreds of thousands of people in the UK who have gone through exactly this experience in the past few years. It is one that no previous generation has experienced, because the blood test that showed James's poor kidney function has only been part of the routine well-man or well-woman testing system since 2005. It has caused a revolution in kidney care. Since it was introduced it has identified around 5 per cent – one in 20 – of the adult population as being in the 'chronic kidney disease' category. This is a far higher number than doctors ever suspected, and has led to big changes in the way we look at kidney problems.

It has also led to treatments to prevent kidneys from deteriorating further, so that most people will never reach the so-called end-stage renal disease that needs dialysis and transplant. So if you have been shocked by the revelation that your kidneys aren't working as well as they should, take great comfort in the fact that we know so much more than we used to about how to look after them, and how to keep them working as efficiently as they can. There is an optimistic 'feel' about chronic kidney disease today, and this book reflects it.

The book explains how our kidneys work in health, why they might start to fail and the consequences of failure. It uses the experience of some of my own patients, in hospital and in general practice, as examples of the ways in which kidney diseases arise, and how they can be treated today.

Most people with moderate kidney disease have their problems managed by their own family doctors, and that is the book's main emphasis. Looking after you involves, for us doctors, a host of aspects apart from prescribing medicines. To begin with, keeping you healthy involves you understanding what happens when your kidneys begin to fail, and what you can do yourself to keep them as healthy as possible. For us doctors, this means giving guidance on how you should live, as well as on the choice of treatments that you face. For you, as a 'kidney patient', taking advice on diet, exercise and lifestyle can be crucial – just as crucial as it is for people with diabetes, heart disease and high blood pressure. So I have spent several chapters on your priorities for keeping well.

For most people diagnosed as having 'moderate chronic kidney disease' the main risk is not that you may eventually have to go on dialysis. If you have been told that you are in this category, then, like James, you are very unlikely ever to reach that advanced stage. On the other hand you are at higher risk than usual of developing high blood pressure, and its main complications of stroke and heart attack. So your doctor's priority for you is to make sure your blood pressure stays low. Simply by doing this you can keep your long-term risks to a minimum. The chapter on blood pressure and prevention of stroke and heart attack is essential reading for everyone with kidney problems (see Chapters 6 and 7).

What you eat, how you exercise, avoiding tobacco and keeping your alcohol intake at reasonable levels all matter more for you than for people with 'healthy' kidneys. Long experience as a general practitioner (GP) has convinced me that repetition of the good health messages is never wasted – so there are chapters on these messages, too.

You will have gathered from this introduction that managing your kidneys won't be simple, so I have taken care in particular in writing Chapter 7, on prescription medicines. When we consider prescription medicines for our kidney patients, we have to obey defined guidelines. The drugs we use to lower blood pressure in kidney patients, for example, are different from those we choose for other patients. Much depends on where the drugs act in the kidneys and on whether they harm or improve the way the kidneys work. That's not easy to explain in non-medical terms, but I've tried to do it so that you can understand fully just why you should be careful to take your medicines as advised. Chapter 7 describes the way in which drugs work in kidney disease and describes those drugs that we most often use, and why.

Although the main premise of this book is that most people with kidney disease will never deteriorate enough to need dialysis, it's inevitable that a few will. So I have included a chapter on kidney dialysis and transplant, based on the experience of the renal unit at Crosshouse Hospital, Kilmarnock, in Ayrshire, Scotland. When I was asked to write this book I spent some time with the doctors, staff and patients at the unit. It is a superb example of the best that the NHS in the UK can offer. Chapter 13 is about my experience there and my interview with Dr Mark MacGregor, its director. I owe Dr MacGregor a huge debt of gratitude for his advice.

Finally, several organizations exist to help kidney patients. They are described and listed at the end of the book (see pp. 112–13). Anyone with kidney disease should be in touch with these organizations: they are a great resource and support. They produce publications on kidney disease that you should also read: where I have drawn on them for information I have given the references, so that you can read them for yourself.

1

The kidneys: where they are and what they do

If you have chronic kidney disease or care for someone with it, you need to know what a normal kidney does and how it does it. Once you know the essentials you will have a better understanding of what can go wrong and how it can be corrected or managed. Such knowledge lets you take part in the decisions that are made on your behalf. That's one of the big changes for the better in my medical lifetime. We now expect our patients to know a lot more about their illnesses and are happy to share the reasons for treatments with you. It makes for much more satisfaction for doctor, carers and patients.

So here goes with the anatomy, physiology and biochemistry of the kidneys! Please don't be put off or skip this chapter, as it is the basis on which the rest of the book depends.

Your kidneys – where they are

Everyone knows what shape kidneys are. We talk of kidney-shaped swimming pools and of kidney beans, and most of us have seen calves' kidneys on a plate. (I must say here that when as a boy I heard what they did, I lost my taste for them.) Those of us who have had a kidney infection have the added, though unwelcome, bonus of knowing precisely where they are. The pain of a kidney infection is precisely sited in the angle between the spine and the ribs beneath the long back muscles that run down the side of the spine.

With a few rare exceptions, we have two kidneys, one on each side of the spine. The one on the right nestles behind the liver, the one on the left behind the bowel and the spleen (Figure 1). Things can – thankfully rarely – go wrong in our development in

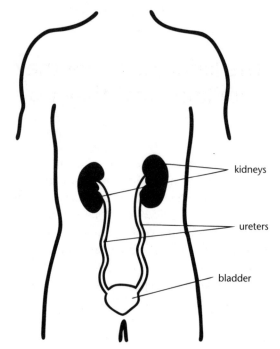

kidneys

ureters

bladder

Figure 1 The position of the kidneys in the body

the womb, so that a few people are born with a 'horseshoe' kidney, in which the two kidneys are joined in the middle across the front of the spine. Others may have a 'duplex' kidney, in which there are two kidneys on one side. I only mention them here because the discovery of a horseshoe or duplex kidney later in life can be a life-saver. I'll come back to them in Chapter 4.

A normal kidney is the size of the palm of a man's hand. It fits snugly in front of the lower edge of the diaphragm, the sheet of muscle that separates the abdomen from the chest. Doctors feel for your kidneys by asking you to lie on your back and to relax the back muscles. They pass the right hand under the ribs and feel with the flat surface of the fingers for the lower 'pole' of the kidneys sliding down below the bottom rib as you breathe in. If you have a kidney infection, firm pressure on that spot as you inhale will make you yelp. It's easier to feel the right kidney because it's slightly lower than the left one, owing to its position below the liver.

The kidneys get their blood supply from arteries – the renal arteries, which arise directly from the aorta, the main artery in the abdomen. There is usually a single renal artery on each side. However, about a quarter of all kidneys have more than one artery feeding them. This isn't a disadvantage until the person needs a transplant, when the surgeon has to match up the new kidney with the 'old' arteries. But that's the surgeon's problem, not yours. Obviously, to make the circulation complete, there is a renal vein companion to the artery. (Arteries take blood from the heart to an organ, and veins remove the blood from an organ and take it back to the heart, from where it flows to the lungs.)

Also leaving the kidneys are the ureters, which carry the urine that has been formed by the kidneys down into the bladder, from where it can be expelled.

What they do

Your kidneys have three main purposes. The first is the one you surely already know about – the production of urine, the main carrier of biochemical waste materials from your body.

You may have an idea of the second, too – the control of the overall amount of water in your body. Put bluntly, you pass less urine when you are dehydrated (you may have been out too long in the sun, or have been running in an exhausting race), and you pass more when you have been drinking too much fluid. The kidneys, by detecting the amount of water in your bodily fluids and circulation, will control their urine output to keep your body water levels in normal limits. Along with the body's water levels, the kidneys also control the amounts of 'electrolytes' in the blood. These include such chemicals as sodium, potassium, magnesium, chloride, phosphate and bicarbonate, all of which are essential substances that must be kept within narrow limits in the blood. There is more about them later, when we come to eating habits and drug treatments (see Chapter 12).

The third function of the kidneys is to control your blood pressure. I describe how they do that in Chapter 2. It is enough to know now that normal kidneys keep your blood pressure within fairly narrow limits. When they start to fail, the blood pressure tends to rise. A rising blood pressure accelerates the progress of damage in a failing kidney: keeping it within the low normal range greatly slows that progression. Which is why we take great care to keep your blood pressure as low as possible.

How they do it

This is the fascinating bit. Each of our kidneys is made up of around a million nephrons. A nephron is a tube (described as a 'tubule' in the textbooks) between 20 and 50 microns wide (a micron is a thousandth of a millimetre) and 50 millimetres long (Figure 2). At one end is a cup-shaped structure, the glomerulus, and the other end joins up with all the other nephron tubes to produce the 'collecting duct' that eventually becomes the ureter, which carries the urine away from the kidney to the bladder.

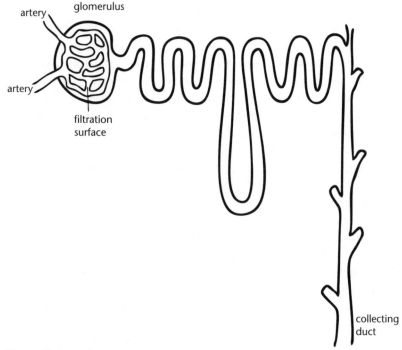

Figure 2 A nephron

The medical textbooks wax lyrical about the structure of the kidney. I love the way H. E. de Wardener, who was the Professor of Medicine at Charing Cross Medical School in London, described it in his classic book *The Kidney* in 1967. 'The total length of the tubules', he writes, 'in the two kidneys is about 70 miles, or more than the distance between London and Brighton.' I have often wondered how he worked that out. However, the description does serve its purpose, for it shows what a huge surface area the kidney has for dealing with the interchange of fluids between blood and urine – and that explains, in part, how we have a massive spare capacity for dealing with kidney problems when they arise. One of the reasons that James didn't know his kidneys weren't working properly is that they have such a lot of spare capacity for dealing with the body's fluids that more than three-quarters of the nephrons must have stopped working before their owner will start to develop obvious symptoms.

To explain how each nephron works, let's start with the glomerulus.

The glomerulus and its tubule

Our million or so (give or take a few) glomeruli are where waste products, plus a lot of water and mineral salts, are actively expressed out of the blood into the start of the tubules. Within each glomerulus is a bunch of capillaries (strictly they are tiny arteries, or 'arterioles') around which lies the 'cup' – the collecting area – of the beginning of the tubule that belongs to that glomerulus. Again, Professor de Wardener comes up trumps with his calculations. He writes that 'the total surface area of the glomerular capillaries in the two human kidneys is about 1.5 square metres – the size, if you prefer it, of a large drawing board or hearth rug.' I'm intrigued as to how he came to that conclusion, too.

In normal kidneys the surfaces of the arterioles and the tubule cells are a single layer thick, making it as easy as possible for water and chemicals to flow through them. It is only when the kidneys are inflamed – either through infection or through problems with the immune system – that they may thicken, which makes the flow of fluids across them more difficult. When that happens, and you have lost a lot of your glomeruli (usually more than 70 per cent of them need to be lost to make much difference), you will start to pass less urine than you used to.

It's enough to state here that the glomeruli are the sites where the blood gives up its waste products as well as a lot of extra water and electrolytes. The glomeruli form much more urine than you actually pass. We measure how well the glomeruli are doing by calculating, from the results of blood tests, the 'estimated glomerular filtration rate' or eGFR. You will probably have heard about it already from your doctor. It's a crucial assessment of your kidney's ability to produce urine from the circulating blood.

The so-called 'normal' eGFR (which I'll go into later) is around 100 millilitres per minute (ml/minute). This means that the glomeruli are passing 100 ml of fluid from the capillaries (the bloodstream) into the tubules every minute. Over a day that would be 180 litres of fluid entering the tubules. The job of the tubules (remember that they are 50 millimetres long) is to make sure that you 'suck back' most of the water and the electrolytes in that fluid, so as to keep your body's overall water and electrolyte balance perfect. In the mean time they must retain all the materials that your body needs to excrete, so that these materials can be passed on into the ureters and bladder.

As we pass only around 1.5 litres of urine each day, the tubules must be returning around 178 litres to the circulation – leaving only that 1.5 litres to be excreted as urine.

It's an easy step to understand from this that when the tubules go wrong, and they can no longer take back the needed water, you will start to pass much more fluid in the urine than normal. This leads, in some forms of kidney failure, to you passing more urine and needing to pass urine more often, even at night. It also leads to problems with your electrolyte balance (remember sodium, potassium, chloride, bicarbonate and phosphate?). If you are leaking too much fluid, you may be losing too much of them, too. How doctors detect and correct such imbalances is covered in the later chapters on kidney disease and its management.

Crucial to both the glomeruli and the tubules is their blood supply. The blood vessels that serve the glomeruli are unique, in that they retain the muscle structure of arteries even after they have left the glomeruli to pass on to the rest of the kidney. Strictly, they do not become veins, which have little ability to narrow, as happens with blood vessels in all other parts of the body. That means that they are able to narrow and 'close off' either before they reach the glomeruli (so that each glomerulus is 'starved' of its circulation and can't work) or after they have gone through the glomerulus, causing back-pressure on the delicate structures within it. If that happens throughout the kidneys, the glomeruli can be badly damaged by the extra pressure. As some blood-pressure-lowering drugs act specifically on these 'efferent' vessels (the ones leaving the glomeruli), we have to choose treatment with great care in patients with both high blood pressure and failing kidneys. There is more about this later, in the chapter on drug treatment (see Chapter 7).

So the message is becoming confusing already. Loss of glomeruli leads eventually to you passing less urine than normal: problems with your tubules usually leads to you passing more urine. And although raised blood pressure is common in kidney disease, not all drugs that lower blood pressure in people with normal kidneys are helpful in people with renal failure. Some may even be harmful.

The tubules also have another, perhaps surprising, function. Around them are cells that detect how much oxygen there is in your blood. If it is less than it should be, these cells send a chemical 'messenger' in the circulation to the bone marrow, which responds by making extra red blood cells. (Red cells carry oxygen from the lungs to the tissues and organs.) The messenger is called erythropoietin – meaning, in Greek, 'the substance that makes red' – or EPO. When the kidneys start to fail, the tubules do not respond normally to a lack of oxygen, not enough red cells are produced, and you become anaemic. Happily we can now supply EPO on prescription for people with this form of anaemia: this is described in more detail on p. 33.

Blood pressure control

On top of all this fine tuning of our body fluids and our red blood cells, the kidneys have another crucial function – to keep our blood pressure within normal limits. This is so crucial to your management of your kidney disease that I've given it a separate chapter.

2

Your kidneys and your blood pressure: what you need to know

Once you get into the routine of being a 'kidney patient', your doctor will take a particular interest in your blood pressure. You might be forgiven for thinking at times that it seems to matter more to your medical team than your kidneys themselves. In fact, you can survive for years with failing kidneys. The 2007 summer issue of the excellent *Kidney Life*, the magazine of the National Kidney Federation, highlights two longstanding 'kidney patients'.

Peter Leslie is still well and enjoying himself after his kidney transplant. There's nothing surprising about that, you might think. Well…he received his new kidney in Belfast in August 1965, 42 years before his interview in *Kidney Life*. Since the transplant Peter has married, had two daughters and a son, and now he and his wife Peggy have five grandchildren. He worked full time until he retired in 1990. He told *Kidney Life* staff that he still has an excellent blood pressure and kidney function.

Then there is Brian Tocher, featured in the same edition. In 2007 he had been on dialysis for 33 years, and is currently attending the dialysis unit in Charing Cross Hospital, in London. Brian has written a book on his time with renal failure, in which he advises readers on how to stick to the renal diet and the fluid restriction necessary for dialysis patients. Details of how to order his book, *Chronic Kidney Failure: Treatment and Diet*, are available from the National Kidney Federation website (see Useful Addresses, p. 112).

My point in mentioning Peter and Brian (and they are by no means unique) is that they have survived many years with end-stage kidney failure – so the failure itself is not what is likely to kill you. Their main reason for their continuing long lives is good control of their blood pressure. I'll take a few paragraphs to explain why, so that you understand why your doctors are so keen to keep your blood pressure under control.

Normal blood vessels, and in particular the arteries that carry blood from your heart to your organs and tissues, are smooth-lined tubes through which the blood flows without hindrance or eddy currents, like the water supply to your house. Their walls are elastic, so that they expand to cope with extra flow, and relax when you rest. They are also muscular, so that they can push the blood onwards in concert with the heartbeat and pulse.

There are two components of the blood pressure – the systolic pressure and the diastolic pressure. The systolic pressure is the pressure exerted on the blood by the beat of the heart. When the lower chambers of the heart – the ventricles – contract, they push the blood into the arteries, and the pressure of that 'push' (medically, the term is systole) is the systolic pressure. When the ventricles relax and expand with the flow of blood into them from the atria (the two upper chambers) above them, this is diastole. In diastole, the valves leading from the ventricles into the arteries close off to prevent the blood from flowing back into the heart from the arteries, and the forward pressure of the blood is maintained by the tension in the artery walls – this pressure is the diastolic pressure.

So when we take the blood pressure we note it down as two figures – the systolic pressure and the diastolic pressure. They are measured in millimetres of mercury (mmHg), and the two figures are separated by a forward slash. So a person with a systolic pressure of 120mmHg and a diastolic pressure of 80mmHg would be noted as having a blood pressure of 120/80. (The systolic pressure is always higher than the diastolic, and it is always given first.)

Normally, your blood pressure remains steady within quite a narrow range. When you exercise or are under stress, it goes up, but when you lie back, rest and relax, it should fall again. Only when the blood pressure remains well above normal when you are in a relaxed physical and mental state are you considered to have high blood pressure, or hypertension.

If your blood pressure remains in the normal range throughout your life, then your arteries tend to remain healthy, with smooth surfaces over which the blood can flow without turbulence. If the blood pressure rises, the structure of the arterial walls has to change to cope with the extra strain on them. They become more muscular and they lose some of their elasticity, and, in the process of thickening, their diameter narrows, so that there is less room in which the blood can flow. Think of gripping a hosepipe hard, and feel the extra pressure under which the water is flowing, and you will get the idea.

If the arteries become narrower, the heart needs to pump harder to force the blood through them, and that raises the systolic pressure. But the narrowing has another effect, too. If it is due to muscle thickening, then the smaller arteries exert more force on their contents, and this explains the rise in diastolic pressure. If the high blood pressure persists, then a vicious circle starts, with the heart beating ever harder, and the arteries responding with more thickening, so that the systolic, then the diastolic, pressures continue to rise.

Mechanisms by which the kidneys can contribute to hypertension

What have the kidneys to do with this process? They are intimately connected with rising blood pressure in four fundamental ways.

Increased body fluids and sodium levels

The first is an increase in your total body fluids – what doctors call the extracellular volume. This happens in early kidney failure because one of the first difficulties the kidneys have is the ability to excrete the electrolyte sodium (which is found in ordinary salt, along with chloride). If we retain too much sodium in our bodies, we have to retain extra fluid to keep our sodium levels correct, and that means our heart has extra fluid to pump around the body. So the systolic pressure rises to cope with the extra load. One of the initial treatments of such kidney problems is to give a diuretic drug that will help the kidneys to remove the extra sodium and the water overload. I'll come to diuretics later in Chapter 7, on drug treatments, but you will surely be familiar with some of the names, such as bendroflumethiazide and furosemide.

Renin

The second, and probably more important, cause of hypertension in kidney failure is a hormone called renin. Renin is produced in normal kidneys as part of a mechanism to maintain blood pressure when it falls too far. It's important for you to understand it, because your treatment may depend on drugs that block the renin mechanisms, and if you know why you are being prescribed them, you will be more comfortable about their use.

In normal health, when the blood pressure falls, as in sleep, the kidneys secrete renin into the bloodstream. The kidneys possess cells that monitor the pressure of the blood flowing through the renal arteries: their automatic reaction to lowered blood pressure is to produce renin. When the renin reaches the bloodstream it sets off a chain of chemical reactions, the final link in which is another chemical called angiotensin. The effect of angiotensin on the small blood vessels in the limbs – and also in the glomeruli – is to make them narrow (a process known as vasoconstriction). In the normal state, with normal kidneys and normal blood pressure, just enough angiotensin is formed from renin to bring a low blood pressure back up into the normal range.

Sadly, once the kidneys have started to fail, they produce more renin than normal (probably in an effort to increase poor blood flow through the glomeruli), and the blood pressure rises constantly. Another vicious circle starts. The more renin the kidney produces, the higher is the blood pressure, and the higher the blood pressure the more damage it wreaks on the delicate blood vessels in the kidneys. The more damaged the kidney becomes, the more renin it produces, and the circle is cranked up another notch.

Knowledge of this biochemical mechanism has led to the development of drugs that interrupt this circle. We can use drugs called angiotensin converting enzyme inhibitors (ACE inhibitors) or angiotensin-2 blockers (AT2 blockers) to prevent the formation of angiotensin by renin. They have the double benefit of lowering blood pressure and protecting the kidneys from further damage. They are described in more detail in Chapter 7.

The adrenal glands

Renin has yet another effect. It also acts on the adrenal glands, which lie across the upper surface of the kidneys. The adrenal glands respond to renin by producing another hormone, aldosterone, which causes the kidneys to retain extra water and sodium, and by doing so, they raise the blood pressure further. We can use aldosterone antagonists to block this action, too.

The sympathetic nervous system

If three mechanisms to push up the blood pressure aren't enough, there is a fourth one, which can be very important in people with kidney problems. All arteries are controlled by the sympathetic nervous system, a network of nerves that, when stimulated, cause the muscles in the artery walls to contract. This muscle contraction causes the arteries to narrow, just like that grip around a hosepipe mentioned earlier. The kidneys are no exception: they are supplied by nerves running alongside their arteries. We know that the arteries in some people with kidney failure over-react to the sympathetic 'message', and that their arteries, again especially the ones supplying the glomeruli, are in a state of near-permanent constriction. This, too, is damaging to the glomeruli and may be yet another reason for the high blood pressure and the progressive kidney failure. For these people, the choice of drug could well be a type of sympathetic blocker drug known to doctors as an 'alpha-blocker'.

Summary

By now you will have begun to understand how complex the choice of drugs for kidney disease can be, and why your doctors have a set of guidelines, worked out by the country's experts, that they use for prescribing for kidney patients. I'll go into these drugs in more detail later in the book (see Chapter 7).

Controlling your blood pressure is one of the most important aspects of your treatment as a patient with moderate kidney disease. The lower your blood pressure is within the normal range, the better are your prospects of keeping your kidneys as healthy as they can be. Your doctor will have several ways of achieving this, with drugs such as diuretics, ACE inhibitors or AT2 blockers, aldosterone inhibitors and perhaps other drugs (see Chapter 7). Your contribution to this care is to take your chosen treatment assiduously, treating it with the same importance as someone with diabetes would their insulin.

But you mustn't depend on the drugs alone. You must follow a lifestyle that will also protect your kidneys and lower your blood pressure. The ways in which you can do this are explained in the next few chapters, after I have described some typical case histories of patients, drawn from my own experience in general practice and from my early years as a hospital doctor.

If you would like to know more about high blood pressure and how you and your medical team can work together to control it, please read *Living with High Blood Pressure*, another of my Sheldon Press books.

I wish I could write that this chapter contains all you need to know about your risks from hypertension, but it doesn't. There is a companion problem to high blood pressure that you also need to know all about if you are to take best care of your kidneys, and that is atheroma. The next chapter is about atheroma, and why you must fight it with just as much will as you tackle hypertension.

3

Atheroma: your kidneys, your heart and your brain

When we are children, the inner linings of our heart and arteries – the surface that is in contact with our blood – are smooth, and the walls of the heart and arteries are muscular and elastic. The blood flows remarkably smoothly through them, without any turbulence.

Sadly, as we grow older, this changes. Fatty deposits start to be laid down in the walls of our arteries. The more fat our bloodstream carries around with it, the more fatty deposits there are. The process starts early. American doctors examining the bodies of young soldiers killed in the Korean War were astonished by the extent of the fatty degeneration in their aortas – the main artery leaving the heart to supply the head, chest, abdomen and limbs. There were even fatty streaks in the young men's coronary arteries, which supply the heart muscle itself. These findings led to the first American efforts to prevent heart disease.

This laying-down of fats in the walls of arteries has a name – atheroma. It is derived from the ancient Greek word for porridge, because the deposits have the look and consistency of blobs of porridge. It's important to remember that this is nothing to do with 'hardening of the arteries', in which the arteries stiffen as the elastic cells in the walls become more fibrous. That is a natural development of old age and a completely separate thing from atheroma.

Deposits – or to use the medical name, plaques – of atheroma appear in the arteries from childhood onwards. The number and size of these plaques are closely related to two properties of the circulation – the pressure within the blood vessels and the level of fats (or 'lipids') in the blood. The best known fat is cholesterol, and it can't have escaped you, unless you have been living on a desert island alone and without a radio for the past 30 years, that the higher your cholesterol level, the higher your chances are of a heart attack or stroke. It also can't have escaped you that living a lifestyle that lowers your cholesterol, along with taking cholesterol-lowering drugs, will help you avoid or at least postpone such catastrophes.

What has this to do with your kidney disease? Actually, quite a lot, although the experts did debate the issue for years before they came to solid conclusions about the links between moderate chronic kidney disease, atheroma, and a raised risk of heart attack or stroke.

John C. Van Stone, Professor of Medicine at the University of Missouri in Columbia, Missouri, wrote about this in 1983 in his book *Dialysis and the Treatment of Renal Insufficiency*. Commenting on the increase in deaths due to heart attacks and strokes in dialysis patients, he noted that he was sure that the fundamental problem was their hypertension. Their constant exposure to high blood pressure, he wrote, was the main reason for the 'accelerated atheroma' that underlay their sudden deaths. Only when there was a history of hypertension in a patient was there also evidence of atheroma severe enough to shorten life. Kidney patients with normal blood pressure were no more at risk of heart attack or stroke than people of the same age and sex without kidney disease.

The esteemed professor's main point, therefore, was that for people on dialysis the blood cholesterol didn't really matter as long as their blood pressures could be kept in the low normal range.

We are not so sure about this today. Professor Van Stone was not seeing patients with milder kidney disease – people who would never have to come to him for dialysis or transplant. Today, if you have been told you have moderate renal failure, you will be advised very firmly that your main future health problem will not lie in your kidney failure, but in your higher than average risk of heart attack and stroke. You will be told equally firmly that there are three main causes of heart attack and stroke – hypertension, a high blood cholesterol level and smoking.

Why has there been such a change in opinion? Twenty or 25 years ago, when Professor Van Stone was writing, he (and all other doctors practising at the time) didn't know the true extent of mild and moderate kidney disease in the population. More importantly, we didn't know its relevance to atheroma and consequently to heart attack and stroke. What brought about the change in thinking was our routine use of more sophisticated tests and measurements to find out who, among our 'healthy' patients, actually had a time bomb ticking in their kidneys. Only when we began to use these tests did we realize the significance of moderate kidney disease. There was mounting evidence that people like James, described in the Introduction (see p. ix), have moderate kidney disease because they have atheroma. It is the fatty degeneration in their arteries that is the main cause of their poor kidney function, and it is a 'red flag' indicating that they have to try to reverse it. This is clearly a separate aim, in addition to lowering their blood pressures. They must also attend to their cholesterol levels.

The proposition is straightforward. I've already explained how important the arteries that supply the kidneys are for the health of the glomeruli. We need perfect blood flow through our million or so glomeruli, so that they can produce the 'filtrate' of 180 litres a day (about 100 ml/minute), and perfect blood flow through the area of our tubules, to make sure that they are doing their job of 'sucking back' all but a litre and a half of this filtrate. If the arteries that lead to the kidneys and the arteries within the kidneys are damaged by atheroma, these two vital components of our kidney function will go wrong, slowly but surely. Remember, too, that the vessels that enter and leave the glomeruli have the structure of small arteries – making them particularly susceptible to atheroma.

Happily, we know a lot about how to treat, arrest and even, to some extent, to reverse, the progression of atheroma in arteries. Our knowledge has come from hundreds of studies in people at risk of heart disease, but it is equally relevant to kidney function. And because people with moderate kidney disease are particularly susceptible to heart disease and stroke, all the advice we give to heart patients about keeping their arteries healthy also applies just as much to kidney patients.

By now you are getting the message that much of your future treatment is largely up to you. Your doctors can give you advice, but it is your obligation, for the sake of your future health, to take it. That's why much of this book is about your future lifestyle, rather than what your doctors can do for you. All the advice on healthy living given to people with normal kidneys applies even more to you as a kidney patient.

If you do follow the advice to the letter, you will hugely improve your chances of avoiding not only progressive kidney disease, but heart disease and the very real prospect of stroke – because the arteries in the brain are just as susceptible to atheroma as those in the kidneys and the heart.

But before we get on to lifestyle, the next chapter deals with what happens when the kidneys go wrong. I've written it using examples of patients, most of them fairly typical of their types of kidney disease, whom I have looked after over the years. You may recognize someone like yourself among them.

4

When the kidneys start to fail: a few case histories

Mild chronic kidney disease – James

We mentioned James earlier. In his 60s, he was found at his well-man check to have moderate chronic kidney failure. He had had no symptoms, and he was shocked to discover that he had a problem at all, far less a serious disease such as kidney failure. Naturally he wanted to know from his doctor how the diagnosis had been arrived at, and what he could do about it.

Estimated glomerular filtration rate

His doctor (me, in fact) explained that the blood test that had highlighted his kidney problem was his eGFR. The eGFR is calculated from the level in the blood of a waste substance called creatinine, using a formula that combines his height and weight (his body mass index, or BMI). James is 1.75 metres (5 feet 9 inches) tall and weighs 76 kilograms (12 stone), so that his BMI was in the normal range – he wasn't obese.

His eGFR was calculated as 45 ml/minute – his glomeruli were processing about 85 litres of fluid per day instead of the usual 180. This was quite a shock for me, as well as for him, because it was much lower than would be expected for his age and put him in the middle of stage 3 chronic renal failure. Glomerular filtration does drop off with age naturally, but certainly not as far as that.

The tables for eGFR are fairly simple. We assume normal is around 100 millilitres/minute. Between 80 and 100 we consider to indicate very minor kidney deterioration, or stage 1 chronic kidney disease. Stage 2 is defined as between 60 and 80. We don't consider any reading above 60 as indicating kidney problems that need serious attention, so that most hospital laboratories don't bother to give a figure if the eGFR is above 60. It is just reported as '>60 mil-lilitres/minute', and nothing more is done about it.

It is only when the eGFR dips below 60 that we consider that the patient is in the 'kidney risk' category. This is stage 3 chronic kidney disease, and is reported as 'moderate loss of kidney function' for regular follow-up.

Moderate kidney function loss, however, isn't yet kidney failure. We don't make that diagnosis until the eGFR drops below 30 milli-litres/minute: by then you have lost more than two-thirds of your nephrons and you are having difficulty in controlling the balance of your water and electrolytes. You may also be losing protein in the urine, and are heading – possibly, but not inevitably – towards the need for dialysis.

At 15 millilitres/minute and below, you are in end-stage renal failure, and are almost certainly looking at dialysis and the trans-plant waiting list.

Blood creatinine and urea levels

James wasn't anywhere near kidney failure, but was, on the basis of that first eGFR, well into stage 3 chronic kidney disease (let's call it CKD), and that needed an explanation. Naturally, on receiving this result, I called him in to talk about it.

During the conversation I explained that the test result depended largely on his blood level of creatinine. Creatinine is a waste product from the breakdown of proteins in the body – mainly from muscles. Why do we break down our muscles? It is a normal result of our daily metabolism. Throughout our lives we are constantly building up our tissues and organs, and removing the waste products from them. It is a matter of balances. Each tissue has a 'turnover' time, in which we replenish old cells that have come to their 'sell-by' date with new ones, and excrete the waste products that have built up in them. Cells with the fastest turnover – a few hours – include the lining cells of our gut and bone marrow cells. Bone cells and red blood cells have a much slower turnover time of several weeks.

Muscle cells are in between. In normal living there is a steady, constant flow of creatinine from them into the bloodstream, which has to be dealt with by the kidneys. If the kidneys are working to full capacity, the levels of creatinine in the blood remain within a normal range, usually around 100 micromoles/litre. If the kidneys are not working efficiently, then they cannot 'clear' as much creatinine from the blood, so that its level in the blood rises. We think of the creatinine level as rising above the normal range when it reaches about 115 micromoles/litre, and we diagnose significant kidney failure when it rises above 200. James's creatinine had been reported as 125, which was slightly worrying.

Kidney function blood tests also measure the level of another waste product, urea. Urea is produced as the breakdown product of proteins in many other organs and tissues, and rising blood levels of urea, like rising blood levels of creatinine, are a signal that the kidneys aren't working correctly. James's urea was 8 millimoles/litre – as with his creatinine level, a little higher than the normal range.

As I started to explain this to James, he stopped me. He asked if the creatinine level could have been higher on the day of the test because he had run in a local half-marathon race the day before.

I pondered that, and then asked him if he had had plenty to drink on the morning of the test. He replied that because he had been asked not to have breakfast before the test, he had not eaten or drunk anything for about 10 hours.

I decided to do his blood tests again. Running 13 miles would certainly increase muscle breakdown and raise blood creatinine above his usual level, and not drinking enough water before the test would have raised his blood urea – which is quite a good reflection of a state of dehydration. The more dehydrated you are, the higher your blood urea is.

On this second occasion, he hadn't been running the day before, and had had a good breakfast with plenty of fluids. We both waited for the results two days later with keen interest.

He now had an eGFR of 57 and a blood urea of 7.1. The eGFR was still in the stage 3 region of CKD, but it suggested that his kidneys were not as seriously affected as we had thought. The urea level was still marginally above the upper limit of normal, tending to confirm that his kidneys were a little damaged.

We took the new readings as more representative of his kidneys' true state of health. He was still officially diagnosed as having mild CKD, but at this level of eGFR I could tell him that, providing that over the next year or so it did not deteriorate further, he would have very little chance (less than 1 per cent) of going into true renal failure and needing dialysis.

However, we couldn't leave things like that. We needed to know, if possible, why his kidneys were working so poorly, and to take active steps to ensure that they could remain at least at the current level. That meant taking a detailed medical life history and doing a few further tests.

James's adult life had been completely illness-free. He had been extremely lucky. He could remember, however, that when he was about 11 years old his doctor had diagnosed 'pyelitis' and had given him a sulpha drug. He thought that his mother had called it sulphadimidine. He had a good memory of the illness, because it had come precisely at the time of his 11-plus examination, and he had had to take a special test later, because he was too ill to take it with the other children. He remembered pain in his back and a high fever, and the doctor testing his urine. He might have had it once more, about a year later, but he wasn't sure.

Pyelitis is an infection of the collecting tubes of the kidneys, possibly ascending from the bladder. It can be the start of a chronic kidney infection, and may initiate the process of chronic renal failure, but in the absence of more frequent attacks later in teenage and as an adult I thought this was unlikely. After all, that first infection had happened more than 50 years before, and any continuing kidney infection would probably have brought him to the surgery years ago.

The next step was to examine his urine again. It had been tested routinely, using a 'dipstick', at the first visit, and had shown nothing abnormal. We now needed to look at it in more detail, to rule out any serious disease that might cause the kidneys to start to fail. So this time a specimen of urine was sent to the laboratory, to look for microscopic evidence of protein and blood.

Examining the urine for protein and blood

Normally, our urine doesn't contain any measurable protein or blood, as detectable on a dipstick test. The fact that you are reading this book suggests that you don't need me to describe dipsticks. Put simply they are small strips of plastic, on the end of which is paper containing chemicals that change colour when exposed to a particular substance. Typical dipsticks will measure levels of protein, glucose, blood, acetone and nitrite, and will also determine the pH (acidity or alkalinity) and specific density of the urine. In people with kidney disease we are particularly interested in proteinuria (protein in the urine) and haematuria (blood in the urine). Nitrite is sometimes of interest, too, as a high 'score' for it strongly suggests a bacterial infection, which could be in the kidney. Glucose and acetone are of more interest in diabetes.

Proteinuria

Protein is one of the three main constituents of our food, along with fats and carbohydrates. Normal kidneys don't allow protein to filter through the glomeruli into the collecting tubes, so it doesn't appear in any significant amount in the urine if the kidneys are healthy. Proteinuria on a dipstick test strongly suggests a kidney problem, and the more protein you pass per day the worse the problem is. Dipsticks show a range of protein from a 'trace' to +++. Anything more than a trace needs to be investigated further.

Laboratory testing of the urine goes much further than the dipstick. We have already mentioned the blood creatinine level, and how the kidneys filter creatinine out into the urine, so that urine does contain plenty of creatinine. The lab test measures both the amounts of creatinine and of protein in the urine, and calculates the 'protein–creatinine ratio', or PCR. Because James had an eGFR below 60, we needed to know if his PCR was high. A high PCR indicates that the kidney is leaking protein abnormally, and is therefore damaged – a low PCR (under 2) is normal.

However, even if your PCR is above 2, that doesn't necessarily mean that you need to worry. About 5 per cent of all people that are randomly tested at well-man and well-woman clinics have minor proteinuria, and as long as the PCR is below 100, it does not indicate serious kidney disease. However, any rise of PCR above 20 or so needs to be followed, say once a year, to rule out any progression in kidney damage. A PCR above 100 suggests possible progressive kidney disease, especially if the eGFR is below 60.

Haematuria

Around 5 per cent of people pass traces of blood in their urine that can't be detected by the naked eye, and most of the time this is not a problem or a sign of kidney disease. However, if there is other evidence of a renal problem, such as an eGFR below 60, it is routine to send a urine sample to the laboratory for a microscopic examination for blood. A laboratory examination gives more information than a dipstick test. Under microscopy the numbers of red cells are counted and reported as estimates of cells per millilitre of urine. Figures of 50 or more suggest a problem that may need to be referred to a kidney specialist or a urologist, depending on where the doctor thinks the blood may be coming from.

If you can actually see blood in your urine, then the likeliest cause in both men and women is an infection. The urine is routinely sent to the laboratory for culture, to detect the organism responsible and to assess the antibiotics to which it is susceptible. However, if there is any reason to doubt that an infection is the cause, then the problem must be investigated further. Where I work, people with haematuria are sent urgently to the 'one-step' urology clinic. What happens there is described in the case of Michael, the next patient (see p. 25).

James's results

James was fortunate. He had no proteinuria or haematuria, either on dipstick or laboratory testing, so it was assumed that his kidneys, although not working at their full potential, would not be a problem in the foreseeable future. Because there was no proteinuria (his PCR was only 1.5) or haematuria, it was decided that the low eGFR was not due to primary kidney disease, such as a chronic infection or glomerulonephritis (which I go into later in this chapter). The story of pyelitis in James's childhood was almost certainly irrelevant to the present day, and he could be reassured that he was not facing rapidly progressive kidney failure in the future.

However, this was not our main concern. A low eGFR in his early 60s suggested that the circulation of blood to his kidneys was already affected by atheroma, and that although the kidneys themselves were not in danger of failure, this was a sign that his general circulation might also be at risk. He was advised that he was at higher than normal risk of a heart attack or stroke, and that we should help him to reduce it.

When we looked at James's other risk factors for heart disease and stroke we were reasonably happy. He had never smoked, and his regular running – six or so half-marathons a year, and training on four days a week with the local athletic club – has kept him slim and physically fit. He could run up hills without breathlessness or pains in his chest, so we considered that an exercise electrocardiogram (ECG) was probably irrelevant for him. His blood pressure at rest was normal, at 120/80, and his resting pulse rate was, as it often is for an athlete, 60 beats per minute.

We were surprised, however, by his blood cholesterol level. The total cholesterol was 6.9 millimoles/litre, 2.3 millimoles/litre of which was high-density lipoprotein (HDL) cholesterol – the 'protective' type. It made the ratio of total cholesterol to HDL a mere 3.0, well below the figure of 5 that would indicate a problem with blood lipids. It is usual to give advice about lowering cholesterol, with a statin drug to lower it further, whenever we find a total cholesterol above 6 millimoles/litre, but would that be correct for James?

Because the 'good' cholesterol was relatively high, it was decided to leave well alone, simply advise James on healthy living and on how to protect his kidneys, and see what the next year would bring. He was not given a prescription, and he was asked to make an appointment in 3 months' time for follow-up blood tests.

That was 18 months ago. James has had five 3-monthly kidney function tests since that day. His eGFRs have all been around 56–59 ml/minute: his urine has remained clear, his cholesterol levels are unchanged, and his blood pressure has remained normal. It is therefore considered that he has the mildest form of CKD and that he will not need special treatment for it unless the figures change for the worse in the future. He is happy with that and has stopped worrying about his kidneys.

Since my practice started to test for kidney disease in our well-man and well-woman clinics, we have picked up several people with a similar pattern of CKD to James's: in fact, around one in every 20 of our 'normal' patients over 60 years old has turned out to have an eGFR of between 50 and 60, with no other abnormal findings. We have managed their early CKD in the same way as we did for James, and so far none of them has had to have his or her management altered because of any deterioration in kidney function. We are lucky, however, in our patients. They have all followed our advice, and some have changed their lifestyles accordingly when it was needed. None was quite as fit as James, and several have taken up exercise; all the smokers have stopped smoking; and quite a few have lost their excess weight. Happily, none of them has yet needed to take drugs.

Another patient with mild chronic kidney disease and other, related problems – Michael

Michael was not one of our well-man clinic discoveries. He came to us because he wasn't feeling well. It was difficult for him to say exactly what was wrong: he just felt unwell and couldn't pinpoint why. He didn't have his usual energy, he felt tired most of the time and he tended to have hot sweats. He wasn't a man to come to his doctor, he said, but his wife had persuaded him to, because she said he 'was no longer the man she had married'.

That was an intriguing phrase, because they had been married nearly 40 years, and were in their early 60s. Surely it was inevitable that he had changed a bit over the years? The underlying meaning of his wife's statement only became clear after Michael and I had talked for a few minutes. For a few months he had felt uncomfortable in his groins – a feeling of fullness in the side of his scrotum, and a tenderness before and after passing urine. At times he thought his urine was a 'stronger colour' than usual and could even be a shade of red. And for the first time in his life he was having to get up at night to pass urine, mostly just once, but sometimes twice. Not only that, he was spending a lot longer emptying his bladder than he used to. When he had to use a public toilet, for example in a restaurant, he noticed that younger men would come in after him and finish well before him.

However, he hadn't felt that any of these symptoms were worth bringing to me or any of my colleagues. Then, finally the 'no longer the man' phrase was explained. He had been refraining from sex for a few weeks because erections caused him a deep pain in the pelvis. Now I had the real reason for his appointment.

I had to examine him, but I first asked him to pass a urine sample. The dipstick test showed haematuria, as I expected, and nitrite, suggesting an infection. I guessed that it was in the prostate gland, which would explain all of his symptoms, from the discomfort in the groins to the deep pain and the difficulties with sex. A chronic infection would also explain his constant tiredness.

Prostatitis

I talked to him about prostatitis, and prepared to send a urine sample to the laboratory to assess the extent of the infection and, if possible, to discover the organism that was causing it. In the meantime I took blood for renal function tests and measured his blood pressure. The last time he had had his blood pressure taken had been 10 years earlier. It had been normal then, but was now at 170/95mmHg. Finally I asked to do a rectal examination.

His prostate gland was tender and enlarged: it wasn't comfortable for him, but the examination confirmed for me the diagnosis. He needed to start treatment with ciprofloxacin, the standard first-line antibiotic for prostatitis, and to return in a few days for the blood results and another blood pressure check.

Hypertension

He was relieved that at least there was a relatively simple explanation for his symptoms, and that we could put him right. However, it wasn't simple. The antibiotic soon began to settle the groin pain and the discomfort, and the blood began to disappear from the urine. His prostate gland became smaller and less tender, and he was able to pass urine more freely and with more force. There were fewer night visits to the toilet.

However, 3 weeks later there was still blood in his urine. His eGFR was only 51 millilitres/minute, and his total cholesterol level was high, at 8.4 millimoles/litre. The practice nurse had regularly measured his blood pressure since his earlier visit, and it hadn't dropped down into the normal range. It remained at around 160/95.

We had to know where the bleeding had come from. Was it the kidney or the bladder, or was there something more seriously wrong than we had thought with his prostate? We had to rule out cancer at any point along the pathway from the kidney to the bladder and beyond.

Further investigations

Michael was given an urgent appointment at our local urology clinic. He was asked to arrive in the morning and was told that the visit would take 2 hours. He was to bring a urine sample with him.

He first met the consultant, who explained all the tests he would undergo on the day. The consultant examined his abdomen and his rectum, feeling the prostate, then arranged for him to 'go on his travels' for a series of tests and examinations. In quick succession he had an ultrasound examination of his abdomen, an endoscopic examination of his urethra and bladder, and an intravenous urogram. In a urodynamic study he was asked to drink a load of water and to pass urine on to a revolving disc that measured the force and maintenance of the urinary stream. Finally he had another ultrasound examination of the bladder to determine his residual urine volume – the amount of urine left in the bladder after trying to empty it.

At the end of the session, his consultant had all the results.

The prostate examination showed that the gland was benignly enlarged, and was pressing against the lower surface of the bladder. This explained the urinary frequency. The ultrasound examination ruled out any abnormal masses and showed a normal kidney outline on both sides. The intravenous urogram confirmed that his kidneys were working well, with no problem areas – except for a tiny stone in the lower segment of the left one. The urodynamic study confirmed the slight blockage of flow caused by the enlarged prostate, and a 5 millilitre residual volume, which is close to normal.

Management

In one way, these results were as good as could be expected. They ruled out serious kidney disease, and the prostate problem could be treated with drugs that helped to 'shrink' it and to relax the base of the bladder – thereby relieving the pressure and allowing better urine flow. They would ease his sense of urgency to pass urine, and probably help him stay in bed all night.

The small stone in the right kidney helped to explain the continuing haematuria, and also helped to reassure the consultant that there was no need, for the moment, to investigate further. However, he was concerned about the high blood pressure, and asked us, his GPs, to control it by prescribing an antihypertensive agent. The one he favoured was an ACE inhibitor.

Michael was therefore put on tamsulosin for his bladder and lisinopril for his hypertension.

Over the next week or so the blood disappeared from his urine, his blood pressure dropped, and he lost his prostate and bladder symptoms. He hasn't had to get out of bed at night to pass urine and according to his wife he is back to his old self. We didn't inquire too deeply into what she meant, but they are once again a happy couple.

However, that isn't the end of the story. His cholesterol remained high, so he was also asked to review his eating and exercise habits, and he was given, in addition to his other drugs, a statin drug to lower it. Over the next few weeks he developed a troublesome dry cough that clearly was a classical adverse reaction to the ACE inhibitor lisinopril, so this was stopped and an AT2 blocker, irbesartan, was given instead. During all this time the ciprofloxacin was continued to make sure that the last of the prostate infection was cured. The standard course of antibiotics for a prostate infection is much longer than for most other infections – in the UK it is 3 months, in the USA it is continued for 6 months.

After 9 months, Michael no longer has blood in his urine. His blood pressure has come down to 125/80, which is fine for him. His eGFR is still around 55, and as that is a slight improvement on the initial results, we are happy with it. However, he will remain on our follow-up list for kidney function tests and for hypertension management for the rest of his life.

Michael and his wife now go walking (briskly – they have two deerhounds) every day. They eat healthily, according to the practice advice; they don't smoke; and they drink only occasionally. They are model patients. When I see them I wonder how much Michael's improved health is due to his new lifestyle and how much to his drugs. But I won't be taking him off them to find out.

Pre-eclampsia and glomerulonephritis – Karen

I first met Karen when she was 25 years old and just pregnant for the first time. As far as I knew she had not had any serious illness in her childhood, and she certainly seemed healthy. We expected her to have a normal pregnancy, and until about the fifth month she was well and happy. Then her blood pressure started to rise, and a little protein appeared in her urine. This was worrying, as it meant that she had a condition of pregnancy called pre-eclampsia, and needed specialist treatment. She spent most of the next 3 months in hospital resting – this was the standard treatment at the time (it was 30 years ago) – and eventually delivered a beautiful baby girl a month early.

When she returned to my care, it took about 2 months for her blood pressure to settle, but it eventually returned to normal, and she and the baby remained well. For a few years we watched her blood pressure twice a year, and it remained in the normal range. But as she reached 40, it began to climb, so that she had to start long-term treatment for it.

It wasn't easy, because the drugs we had then were diuretics and beta-blockers, and although they kept the blood pressure at a reasonable level, it was never lowered to quite what we wanted. We could manage to keep her systolic pressure at around 145–150 and her diastolic pressure between 85 and 90.

At the age of 50 she had her first test for eGFR. We were shocked to find that it was 42, in the lower reaches of stage 3 CKD. She had no symptoms and did not feel unwell. Her urine showed some protein, and the laboratory result confirmed a PCR of 150. Because of her long history of hypertension, her relatively young age and the high PCR, we asked for a consultant nephrologist's opinion on what we should do next.

It's probably useful here to describe the difference between a nephrologist and a urologist. Nephrologists are renal physicians, who deal specifically with kidney diseases that have to be treated medically. They investigate patients who have been found to have protein in their urine and poor kidney function. They are also in charge of dialysis units, and they look after people who have had renal transplants. Urologists are surgeons who investigate and, when necessary, operate on people suspected of having conditions such as kidney and bladder stones, enlarged prostate glands, and cancers.

Karen's nephrologist took a careful medical history going back to her childhood, spending some time going over the years since then, and finally coming to the present. He examined her, and arranged for an ultrasound scan and a biopsy of one of her kidneys.

The thought of someone putting a needle into her scared Karen, but the consultant was calm and reassuring, and she accepted that it was needed so that we could understand why she was losing so much protein in her urine. It wasn't as bad as she dreaded. He asked her to lie face down with a cushion under her abdomen and her arms above her head. This brings the kidney fairly close to the surface of the back. A small needle delivered some local anaesthetic to the spot, and the biopsy needle was slipped in painlessly to the target. She had been warned beforehand to hold her breath and to expect a 'pop' when the biopsy was being taken. It was done before she knew it, with no discomfort. She was then taken to the day ward to lie down on her back, and was watched over for 6 hours before she went home.

The biopsy confirmed that Karen had extensive damage to her glomeruli, probably because she had had an inflammation of them many years before. The condition is called glomerulonephritis, and it is thought to be an abnormal reaction of the immune system to some 'challenge' (perhaps an infection or some unknown chemical or allergen) that causes the immune system to start to destroy the body's own tissues. The acute illness had long disappeared, but it had left her with kidneys that were slowly deteriorating over the years. It is a process that could eventually, if not slowed or stopped, lead to end-stage renal failure.

We still don't know how to treat the cause of glomerulonephritis or how to reverse its effects, but once we know someone has it we can employ a host of measures to slow its progress and, it is hoped, to keep the kidneys healthy enough to avoid the need for dialysis or transplant.

The first, and most important, step in Karen's case was to make a determined effort to control her blood pressure, and to keep it around 120/80mmHg. As we had been trying to do this for years, it wasn't going to be easy. With help and advice from the nephrologist, she was given an AT2 blocker, irbesartan, rather than a beta-blocker. As she had glomerulonephritis, the obvious reason for her hypertension was that her kidneys were producing too much renin, and a drug like irbesartan would directly block its action. If we could stop the vicious circle described in Chapter 2, in which kidney disease produces high blood pressure and the high blood pressure in turn damages the kidneys to produce more kidney disease, we might be able to arrest her CKD at this point. And as she was not in herself feeling unwell, that would be a satisfactory result.

The decision proved to be the right one. Within a month her blood pressure was down to 125/85mmHg, and within 2 months, it was 120/80mmHg. Her urine contained less protein than before, and her PCR had fallen to below 100. These were encouraging results. Her eGFR has remained around 40 for the last 2 years, and the kidney team are happy that her illness does not seem to be progressing so fast that she will need dialysis in the foreseeable future.

It wasn't the new drug alone, however, that helped to bring down her blood pressure and kept her well. Karen co-operated fully with all her advisers – who included her GP, her nephrologist, her practice nurse, her dietician and even her 30-year-old daughter, who is now a sports adviser and trainer at our local health club and spa. She obeys all the rules for coping with CKD. She is eating sensibly, she exercises regularly, she limits her alcohol intake to fewer than 10 units a week and she does not smoke. She never forgets her blood pressure tablets and she always attends her follow-up appointments. In fact she is a model patient.

Kidney disease caused by earlier radiotherapy – Indira

I often wish that we had met Indira much earlier than we did. She came as a schoolteacher from India as a 35-year-old in 1981. Unusually for an Indian woman she had never married. Happily, soon after she arrived in the UK, she met and married a widower from her own community. He had two sons, and she soon became the perfect stepmother to them. She settled well into British society, and all seemed well.

I met her in 1990, when she came to me complaining of feeling weak and tired all the time. She looked pale and drawn, and my immediate impression was that she was physically ill. Recently – within the previous 2–3 months – she had developed puffy bags under her eyes and swollen ankles, and she was finding that walking up a slope made her breathless. She had no pain. Before examining her I asked about her previous medical history, and I was shocked to learn that in her teenage she had had a hysterectomy for what had been diagnosed as a uterine tumour. The operation had been followed up with radiotherapy to her abdomen.

She knew nothing about the type of tumour or why she had had to have such severe treatment, and when we wrote to her old hospital in India, it turned out that her operation notes had been destroyed years before.

Her infertility, of course, explained why she didn't marry and had made a career as a teacher. But did it also help to explain her illness?

Her puffy eyelids were full of fluid, as were her ankles. Pressing my thumb on her ankles and the top of her feet left a thumb-shaped dimple, indicating that the swelling was retained fluid. Her blood pressure was dangerously high at 210/150mmHg, and her urine was full of protein. In 1990 we didn't have the eGFR test, but we could measure her blood urea level, and this was well into renal failure levels at around 50 millimoles/litre. (The upper limit of normal for urea in the laboratory was 7.5.) At that time we used to measure creatinine clearance, a similar measurement to the eGFR. Hers was only 29, meaning that she had lost nearly three-quarters of what we would consider normal adult kidney capacity.

She was also very anaemic. Her haemoglobin was only 7 grams/litre, around half of what it should have been. Haemoglobin is the pigment that makes blood cells red. It picks up oxygen in the lungs and sheds it in the organs and tissues. Loss of haemoglobin, or anaemia, therefore diminishes the oxygen-carrying capacity of the blood. To compensate for this, the heart has to beat faster to cause what haemoglobin we have left to pass faster round the circulation, and therefore speed up the pick-up rate of oxygen. If we can't compensate fully for the loss of haemoglobin, we feel tired and drained in energy. At a haemoglobin of only 7 grams/litre, Indira couldn't compensate, and she was in a state of being 'tired all the time'.

She needed immediate hospital admission under a nephrologist. At that time the crucial test was an intravenous pyelogram, which involves injecting a dye (that can be seen on X-ray) into a vein and watching its progress through the kidneys. Both her kidneys were about half the usual size, and the dye was passing through much more slowly and in much less concentration than normal.

This brought her treatment as a teenager into sharp focus. The nephrologist concluded that both kidneys had been irretrievably damaged by her radiotherapy, and that they were now undergoing a process of progressive scarring. It would not be possible to reverse this, but the team would do its best to slow it down. He felt that the best we could do for her would be to postpone the time when she would need dialysis, and possibly transplant.

Indira followed her instructions to the letter over the next few years. She needed several antihypertensive drugs to bring down her blood pressure and diuretics to stimulate her kidneys to produce more urine, and she had to restrict her fluid intake. One of her particular problems was that, being a conscientious Hindu, she was vegetarian, and it was difficult for her to adapt to the renal failure diet that she was asked to follow. Her blood potassium and phosphate levels were too high, and she had to cut down severely on fruits and vegetables. For the first time in her life she tasted meat, which until then was anathema to her. However, she recognized that it was essential for her well-being.

She was also one of the first of my patients to receive EPO. The nephrologist assumed, correctly, as it turned out, that her anaemia was the result of a vicious circle. First, the damaged kidneys could not excrete enough urea, so that blood urea levels had risen. Bone marrow is sensitive to a rising blood urea level: it responds by slowing its production of red cells. This leaves the blood with less circulating oxygen capacity. Normal kidneys would detect the low oxygen level and respond by producing EPO. Damaged kidneys like Indira's either can't do this at all or else can't produce enough to stimulate the bone marrow's red cell production, so the anaemia simply gets worse. Giving regular injections of EPO helped to stimulate her marrow enough to raise her haemoglobin to around 10 grams/litre, which made her feel much better. She was no longer 'tired all the time' and started to enjoy life again.

As the years passed, her kidney function worsened, until in 1995 she had to start dialysis. She was trained to use peritoneal dialysis at home, and managed on it very successfully for 4 years, with only the occasional infection. She was even able to go on holiday several times to Cyprus, where the hotel helped to provide the facilities she needed. Her fluids came with her. Finally she had her transplant, and for the first time was able to travel for a holiday to India. Her current eGFR is 57 and her urea level 6.9. Her new kidney has made all the difference to her quality of life. It also makes its own EPO: her haemoglobin is now constantly between 11 and 12 grams/litre, and she feels very happy with it.

A bonus of the transplant has been that we have been able to keep her blood pressure much lower than before. Injecting EPO has one big problem that is difficult to deal with completely. It tends to raise the blood pressure, and even with combinations of antihypertensive drugs, it is difficult to reach the usual target blood pressure. Now that her pressure is under better control we expect Indira's risk of stroke and heart attack to be much less than it was.

I include Indira's case because we can't keep all people with CKD out of dialysis. She was exceptional because her kidney disease was almost certainly doctor-induced. We will never know whether the operation and radiotherapy were justified, but it is a salutary lesson. Today, if a young woman needs radiotherapy for a tumour inside the abdomen, the kidneys are protected by shields and the rays are much more focused on the area that needs treatment, with little, if any, spread to the surrounding tissues. However, she is not alone in having kidney disease that is caused by medical treatment. Mary is another such case.

Analgesic nephropathy – Mary

Mary has had headaches, muscle and joint pains all her life. It's difficult to know why she has them, but they are certainly very real. She has had all sorts of investigations for them, but no diagnosis has ever been made. Her joints show no sign of arthritis on examination, on the usual blood tests or even on X-ray. There is nothing in her skull or scalp to explain her headaches. She has been examined and tested, and sent to various consultants, including a psychiatrist, and none has found a convincing explanation for her pains.

Not surprisingly, she became disillusioned with orthodox medical care and visited osteopaths, chiropractors, herbalists and yoga teachers, but she still had her pains. The only relief she could get from them came from bottles of painkillers. Eventually she was taking every day several paracetamol tablets along with another eight or so ibuprofen tablets, which she bought regularly from the pharmacy. They seemed to ease the pain a little, and she stopped visiting her doctors or her alternative practitioners.

The fact that she had stopped asking for appointments only served to persuade her doctors that her pains must be better, so they did not find it odd that she was no longer a regular weekly visitor.

Then, when she was 55, she fell crossing the street, and was brought in to the health centre with a pain in her left hip. Her doctor found she had a fractured femur (thigh bone) and sent her to hospital, where she needed surgery to repair it. A fractured femur in your 50s, especially in a woman, strongly suggests osteoporosis – loss of minerals such as calcium and of bone-building proteins from the bones.

It is routine, therefore, for everyone with a bone fracture to be tested for osteoporosis and for all its possible causes. When Mary's results came back, they confirmed that she was very low in blood vitamin D levels, and that the bone densities in her wrist, spine and femur were all well into the osteoporosis zone. There was an added surprise. Her eGFR was only 35.

Now that the diagnosis of CKD was made, her orthopaedic surgeon passed her on to the nephrologist. He soon discovered her habit of swallowing large quantities of anti-inflammatory drugs, and asked her to stop them. The two consultants worked together – the orthopaedic surgeon gave her a series of active exercises to do to help with her chronic back pain, and he prescribed medication for her osteoporosis, while the nephrologist guided her on how to live with her CKD.

The results were astonishing. The exercises – designed to stretch her cramped back muscles and to improve her posture – helped for the first time to eradicate her longstanding pain. Stopping the painkillers produced an immediate improvement in her eGFR. Over the next few months it rose into the 50s. There was an extra bonus: her vitamin D levels rose and her bone density improved. She began to look taller and straighter than she had for years.

Why did she improve so much? Another function of the normal kidney, apart from its production of urine, its maintenance of mineral balance, its stimulation of red cell production, and its control of blood pressure, is that it 'activates' vitamin D.

Vitamin D, the kidneys and osteoporosis

Let me digress a little to explain vitamin D and the crucial role that it plays in preventing bone disease. We obtain vitamin D in two ways: from fatty and oily foods, such as fish, vegetable oils and fortified dairy products; and from the action of sunlight on the skin. However, it has to pass through the kidney circulation to be turned into the active vitamin. Once activated (for the technically minded, the kidney turns vitamin D into 1:25-dihydroxy-vitamin D), it can then do its job of driving calcium into the bones to keep them strong. If the kidney fails to activate our circulating vitamin D, then it won't work, and the bones lose their mineral strength. In adults, medically this is called osteomalacia; it is rickets in children. However, it has come to be called popularly osteoporosis. Whatever you call it, when the kidneys deteriorate enough to stop activating vitamin D, you are in danger of sustaining fractures such as Mary's.

Mary probably was more prone than others to develop osteoporosis: her mother, she told us later, had had it in her sixties. Why had she developed it earlier than her mother? One clue lay in her massive consumption of anti-inflammatory drugs over many years. Non-steroidal anti-inflammatory drugs such as ibuprofen and naproxen, taken in high doses over years, can damage the kidneys to produce a syndrome like CKD. Her long-term use of them had produced an 'analgesic nephropathy', the medical term for a kidney damaged by painkillers, and the vitamin D disturbance may have been part of the nephropathy.

Long-term management

Happily, analgesic nephropathy is one form of CKD that is reversible, which is why she responded so well to stopping her drugs.

Mary is now an energetic exerciser. She is another of our CKD patients who has joined the local spa, where her training schedule is overseen by one of our physiotherapists.

Diabetes and kidney disease – Elaine

Elaine developed diabetes when she was 8 years old. She adapted well to the life of several daily insulin injections and regular blood tests, and until she was 17 there were no complications. Then teenage rebellion took over, and she didn't look after herself so strictly. She discovered alcohol and wanted to enjoy herself like all the other teenagers.

For a while, her blood glucose levels weren't as well controlled as before. She had a few mishaps with alcohol, failing to stick to the healthy eating advice, and even missed one or two insulin injections. Once or twice she even ended up in hospital. It took her several months to realize that she was damaging herself, and that she needed to take more care. With the help of her general practice team and her diabetes specialist, she returned to her previous self-discipline.

It isn't clear why, from then on, she started to have CKD. It may have been her straying from the diabetes discipline, or it may have happened anyway, but for the first time, her urine tests were abnormal. There was no protein on the dipstick test, but the lab reported that she had microalbuminuria. This means that the kidneys were leaking protein in microscopic amounts – not enough to show on a dipstick, but enough to say that she was starting to have diabetic nephropathy, a type of CKD associated with diabetes.

Although Elaine's blood pressure was not raised – it remained, as it had for years, at 125/80mmHg – she was asked to take an ACE inhibitor drug, lisinopril. This is a blood pressure-lowering drug (an antihypertensive agent) that prevents the conversion of renin into angiotensin (see Chapter 2). Several studies have shown that blocking angiotensin formation, either with an ACE inhibitor or an AT2 blocker will help to prevent further kidney deterioration, regardless of whether or not the blood pressure is raised.

She has now been taking lisinopril for 2 years. Her eGFR is still above 60, and she still has microalbuminuria, but no dipstick-positive protein. We hope that her kidneys will remain in a healthy state, but she will be followed up for the rest of her life as part of the practice CKD surveillance. She is now a university student and enjoying life without dropping her self-discipline. She regrets her teenage lapse, because she knows it damaged her eyes, as well as her kidneys, but her medical team has worked hard to help her to lose her sense of guilt over it. It is understandable that many youngsters with diabetes kick over the traces in their late teenage years, and it's hardly fair to blame them for it.

Two patients from the past and one from today with immune disorders – Christine, Colin and John

Henoch-Schönlein purpura – Christine

The kidney differs from all other organs in its susceptibility to immune disorders. As a newly qualified doctor working in the Children's Hospital in Birmingham, I remember our despair when we had to admit as emergencies teenagers who had developed acute kidney failure.

Christine was a typical case. About a week earlier she had had a sore throat, which had apparently resolved itself as sore throats do. Then she developed a bright red rash on her legs, with pains in her joints and abdomen. She felt very ill, and was frightened further when she saw that her urine was red.

His doctor knew what it was and sent her in to hospital, with a note to say that there was blood and protein in her urine. We made the diagnosis of Henoch-Schönlein purpura with acute renal failure. The rash, which didn't blanch with pressure on it, turned purple over the next few days and eventually faded to yellow. All we could do was to wait and watch to see if she would recover, because at the time we had no medical regimen that would have made a difference.

Christine was one of the luckier ones. After a week or so, she began to improve, the haematuria became less and the protein almost disappeared from her urine. She felt much better. However, 6 months later, at follow-up, there was still some proteinuria, and her blood pressure was slightly higher than expected for the average 16-year-old. She was on her way to chronic kidney disease.

I often wonder what happened to Christine. She became ill just as dialysis was coming into regular use for patients with CKD. I left the hospital for a career in general practice shortly after I met her, and didn't see her again. Did her kidneys hold out into the era of dialysis, and how did she manage?

Goodpasture's syndrome – Colin

Colin didn't fare so well. At 20 he had just started at university. It was 1968, during the last great influenza pandemic. I was in general practice at the time, and was rushed off my feet looking after hundreds of patients. Colin was one of them. Two days after he caught the flu he suddenly coughed up about half a litre of bright red blood and became extremely breathless. I was called to him as an emergency, and because he had serious sounds of fluid in his chest and his blood pressure was dropping, sent him straight to hospital in a 'blue light' ambulance.

Within 3 days, his chest was a little better, but it became clear that he had kidney problems, too. He had haematuria and proteinuria and his blood tests showed that he was in acute renal failure.

Colin's was a classic case of what was then called Goodpasture's syndrome. Sadly he followed the expected path of the syndrome then: his kidney failure didn't recover, and he died within 2 months.

Management of immune diseases affecting the kidney today – John

Today, thankfully, life is different for people with Henoch-Schönlein purpura and Goodpasture's syndrome. We know now that 'immune complexes' circulating in the blood cause the damage to the kidney. They form in the blood as a consequence of our immune system fighting off 'foreign' proteins, which either derive from infectious agents such as viruses (influenza is typical) or bacteria (such as streptococci – the agent causing a typical sore throat) or from allergens (such as a bee sting, pollen or dusts).

In a typical normal immune reaction, our body forms antibodies to the foreign 'antigens'. They fit together like pieces of a jigsaw,

and the resulting complex neutralizes the illness-producing potential of the 'invader'. However, on extremely rare occasions, the
complex is toxic to the delicate tissues of the nephron. Both the
glomeruli and the tubules become inflamed and, if the reaction is
severe enough, they are eventually destroyed.

This is what happened to Christine and Colin. Their kidneys
were damaged by the immune complexes. In Christine's case they
also damaged the circulation in the skin, causing the rash. In
Colin's case the lungs took the brunt of the attack.

Today, both would have been treated positively, and they would
surely have recovered. They would have their blood 'filtered' free
of the complexes, using special dialysis techniques, and their acute
kidney failure would be reversed.

This is what happened to John, whom a colleague of mine was
asked to see in 2007. He was 25 years old, and had been completely
healthy. He phoned for a visit because he had woken up one
morning feeling awful, unable to get out of bed without excessive
effort and great tiredness. He was still reluctant to ask for help,
however, feeling that it was just 'bad flu', until his wife saw his
rash. It was bright red and covered the bottom half of his body and
legs.

His doctor, seeing the rash, asked about his urine. John then
remarked that it was odd, but he didn't think he had passed any
urine for nearly 24 hours, and he wasn't able to produce a specimen
to order. Recognizing the probability of acute renal failure, his GP
sent him to the local renal unit, where his eGFR was found to be as
low as 7. His PCR was almost 1,000.

John was dialysed and his blood filtered. It took him some weeks
to recover from the episode of acute renal failure, but he is now
doing well. His kidneys have recovered so far that he is now in stage
3 CKD, with an eGFR of around 33. The cause of his acute failure
was never found, and he has been reassured that he is over the
worst. But his outlook isn't yet secure. His doctors are watching to
see if the eGFR can be maintained at his present level, or if it will
start to deteriorate again. For John it is 'wait and see' – but it is a far
better outcome than in the past.

Inherited kidney problems – of horseshoes and cysts

Most people who later develop CKD have started off life with normal kidneys and, to misquote Shakespeare, have had their illness thrust upon them. Some, however, are born with kidney disease in the making. They have inherited abnormal kidneys (Figures 3 and 4).

They may have only one kidney, the other having never developed or having stayed small with very little if any urine-producing capacity. Some may have two kidneys, but they are both on the same side. Others still have a 'horseshoe' kidney, in which there is one large kidney across the upper abdomen. There may be an 'ectopic' kidney, meaning that it is not in the usual site in the angle between the ribs and the spine, but in the pelvis instead. Sometimes the kidneys themselves are normal, but there are two ureters arising from the same kidney: they may join together on the way to the bladder, or enter the bladder separately.

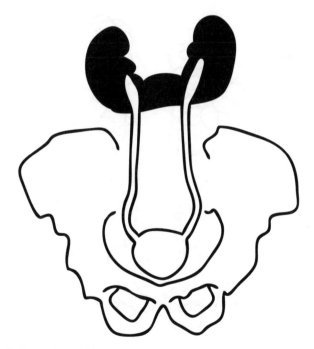

Figure 3 Horseshoe kidney

In all these cases, there is little evidence to suppose that their 'owners' are more likely than others to develop CKD. Some may be more prone to urinary infections, but most of these kidney anomalies are found by accident, when a person is under investigation for another illness. If one kidney is absent, for example, the remaining one usually enlarges to compensate for the loss of its companion, but it is usually as efficient and as healthy as two normal kidneys would be.

According to my old friend Professor de Wardener, in his book, about one in 200 of us go through life with one of these types of anomalous kidney without ever knowing about it.

Polycystic kidneys – Charles

One inherited kidney problem, however, does cause many people grief – polycystic kidneys. Charles's case is fairly typical. Charles was 38 when his polycystic kidneys were diagnosed. His main com-

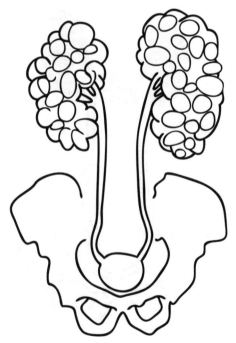

Figure 4 Polycystic kidneys

plaint was that for some months he had felt 'swollen' or 'distended' in his upper abdomen. What brought him to the surgery, however, was that he had fallen playing football with his young son, and he thought that the pain he felt around his lower ribs was much greater than it should have been. He was tender and uncomfortable near the sides of his lower ribs.

His doctor found that his kidneys were surprisingly easy to feel, even without Charles having to breathe in. They felt 'knobbly' and firm. As something was obviously not right, he tested Charles's urine: there was a moderate amount of protein in it. Charles's blood pressure was a little high, at 145/90mmHg, but not at the level one might expect in more severe CKD. And he hadn't experienced any problems passing urine. He didn't need to get up at night to do so, and there was no pain or discomfort related to passing it or afterwards.

There was one clue to the diagnosis. Asked about his family history, Charles thought that an uncle and a great-uncle had died young of 'problems with their kidneys', but he didn't know their diagnoses. His father (the uncle's brother and the great-uncle's nephew) had been killed at 28 in a road accident, so presumably had not survived to an age at which the disease might have been diagnosed.

A urogram showed that Charles had cysts in both kidneys. He was given the diagnosis of inherited polycystic kidney disease, and was put on the practice CKD register. His eGFR was 45, and he was the subject of a long conversation involving the urologist, the nephrologist and the GP. Some of the cysts were large and obviously the cause of his discomfort and pain, so it was decided to decompress them, purely to ease the symptoms. The nephrologist could not reassure him that the operation would relieve his CKD but it did ease his symptoms and allay some of his fears. Having heard that he had cysts in his kidneys he was naturally frightened that they might burst if he exerted himself, despite being reassured that this would not happen.

He was also worried that he might progress to end stage renal failure like his two relatives, but was reassured that, with today's treatments, this could be avoided. He was started on an antihypertensive drug, his high cholesterol (a separate issue from polycystic disease – they are not necessarily related) was treated with a statin drug, and he was placed on 3-monthly follow up.

For the last 2 years his eGFR has remained steady at 45, his proteinuria has remained moderate, with a PCR of around 60, and he is much more comfortable. His kidneys are no larger than they were at the time of diagnosis, and it is assumed that he will be able to live for many years without his condition diving into stage 5 CKD.

Charles's story is typical of most people with polycystic kidneys. Although they are born with the abnormality, it doesn't cause symptoms at least until they reach adulthood and not usually until their late 30s. There is a childhood form, but it seems to be separate from the adult disease and to be inherited in a different way. Technically, the childhood disease is caused by a recessive gene, and it is therefore much rarer than the adult form, which has a dominant genetic inheritance. Both forms of the disease affect both sexes equally, and the family tree, if known, usually has a scattering of cases.

Today, when the diagnosis of polycystic kidneys has been made, we ask close relatives to come in for a check to rule out or confirm the problem. That is how many, if not most, cases are diagnosed, usually before there are symptoms of any sort. It is good to find the condition early, because the patients can then usually go on a regimen in time to arrest or slow the development of CKD.

However, some people with polycystic kidneys slip through the net, and don't appear until they have symptoms. Apart from the abdominal discomfort, bloating and pain that Charles experienced, polycystic kidney disease may initially show itself as a bout of haematuria – the patient finds that he or she is passing red urine – or a kidney infection. Pain on passing urine ('dysuria') along with pain in the back, with fever and sweating, are common 'presenting symptoms'. A diagnosis of pyelitis is made. The rule in pyelitis is that it is unusual in a man: if he has two bouts of it he should be investigated. If there is persisting proteinuria even after the first bout, he should be investigated. Women, because of their anatomy, are more prone to urinary infections than men, but they, too, need investigation if they have more than one kidney infection.

Often all that is needed is a good abdominal examination by the GP: those knobbly kidneys are a 'give-away', as is the presence of measurable protein in the urine. And the day at the urology clinic that is now mandatory for further testing in cases like this will certainly show the cysts, their bulk and their severity.

Occasionally, polycystic kidneys are found only by chance, after a routine well-man or well-woman check has found the combination of higher than normal blood pressure with proteinuria. Interestingly, polycystic kidneys are one cause of CKD that doesn't always raise the blood pressure. It is raised in about three-quarters of cases, and even then the rise is moderate: it is rarely excessive. If a very high blood pressure is found in someone with polycystic kidneys, we will look for another cause for it.

If you have just been given the diagnosis of polycystic kidneys, don't be surprised if your doctor can't give you a clear idea of how your CKD is likely to progress. Some people stay at the same level for years, others tend to progress more rapidly. In the days before dialysis and transplant surgery, according to de Wardener, people lasted around 10 years after the date of diagnosis, but he admits that 'if renal infections are treated promptly some patients live many years without appearing to deteriorate'.

That is the aim of treatment of polycystic kidney disease today. If you have it you will be on a CKD management regimen that aims to extend the years before you will need dialysis or transplant and, if possible, to avoid the need for them completely.

In fact, that is the aim for everyone with CKD. All the patients described in the last few pages were placed on a CKD management regimen. You have probably recognized your own story among them. How they, and you, achieve the aim of the regimen is what the rest of this book is about.

5

Managing stage 3 CKD: the principles

So you have been told that you have CKD. Naturally your immediate thought is: 'Will I die from kidney disease? I've heard and read so many frightening stories about kidney failure, dialysis and transplants that I can't bear to go down that road.'

On the day I'm writing this chapter, in January 2008, the main news is that the British Prime Minister, Gordon Brown, has asked for the routine removal of organs, including, of course, kidneys from all dead bodies except where the person has previously expressed a wish for this not to happen. The reason for this drastic step? That around 1,000 people in the UK are dying each year from kidney failure while waiting for transplants. The present system asking for people to volunteer to allow their organs to be removed after death has not produced nearly enough donations.

It is scary to be told that you have CKD. If I do need a transplant, you think, will there be one for me, or will I be one of the thousand to wait in vain? Is the alternative death from kidney failure?

Please banish these thoughts. The vast majority of people with CKD never reach its end stage, when they need dialysis or transplant. They live normal lives with as little discomfort as their neighbours without kidney disease. To do so, they need to obey the rules, but these rules are only what common sense and a little knowledge about healthy living dictate to us. Everyone, with or without CKD, should follow them. There is just one 'but'. You must be a little stricter than others about your health – because if you are not, you are at higher risk than the rest of the population of suffering from cardiovascular disease – heart attacks and strokes. This higher chance of dying from cardiovascular disease, not ultimate kidney failure, is the real risk for you.

So your aim is to do everything to cut down your risk of heart attack and stroke. In doing so, you will also be improving the health of your kidneys, which is a big bonus. Keeping your circulation healthy not only protects your heart and brain, it protects your kidneys too. I make no apology for devoting the next few chapters to the details of how you can do so.

The three main risks – high blood pressure, high cholesterol and smoking

Look upon your circulation as a closed flexible, elastic tube with a pump (your heart) and auxiliary pumping stations (the muscles in the walls of your arteries) along the way. Imagine such a system as heating your house. If the water pressure is too high, the tubing may crack under the strain and burst. If the lining of the tubing is furred up with deposits of material (say lime scale in a hard-water area), then the water can't flow through it and, without a plumber to remove the deposits, the flow will eventually stop. If the boiler has to work too hard to pump the water through it, it will burst. Or if the pump is neglected, and corrodes, it will break down.

Of course, the analogies are simplistic, but they do bear some thought. High water pressure equates to high blood pressure. The lime scale idea isn't too different from deposits of calcium or cholesterol in the lining of arteries in the heart, brain and kidneys – and it has the same effect of reducing the blood flow through them. It is a good model for what happens in strokes, heart attacks and kidney damage caused by failing oxygen supply to the tissues. And if you neglect your 'pump', you are looking forward to heart failure.

Let's turn to humans. We have mentioned high blood pressure and high cholesterol levels before. They are two of the three main risk factors for cardiovascular disease. The third is smoking. Any one of these risks is bad enough for people with CKD: if you have two, then it is serious. If you admit to all three, and don't want to change, then you should be starting to think of putting your affairs in order. If you still feel the same way after reading the next three chapters, don't bother reading the rest. Other people can't help you unless you are determined to help yourself.

Other risks

There are also subsidiary risks. Having diabetes and CKD puts extra pressure on you. The two together combine to make you at even higher risk of cardiovascular disease. So you need to be in good control of your diabetes as well as your general health. Elaine's story (see p. 37) explains how the combination of CKD and diabetes can be lethal if not managed meticulously.

Being too heavy doesn't help, either. Extra weight puts strain on your heart that complicates its problems. Nor does physical idleness. Exercise is important. We all know how difficult that can be when you are not feeling 'up to it', but do try to follow the advice on exercise when you can. Your kidney team will advise you on how much you can do, for how long and how many times a week.

Then there is eating wisely. If you haven't heard about fruit and vegetables and 'five a day' you must have been on Mars for the past 10 years. What you eat is particularly important if you have CKD, especially if you are getting down towards stage 4, with less than a third of your kidney function left. If that is you, there is a chapter for you, with advice on how to manage your electrolyte and mineral balance (see Chapter 12).

Finally, there is your mental attitude to kidney disease. Understand that you aren't alone. A staggering one in every 20 people over the age of 60 is now thought to have an eGFR below 60 – the criterion that puts them in stage 3 CKD. Obviously that is a far higher proportion of the population than ever reaches the dialysis teams and the transplant lists. In our local general practice of around 1,800 patients, there is one on dialysis, and around 100 with an eGFR below 60. We don't expect more than three or four to get to a stage at which they will need dialysis.

So look on your CKD as an inconvenience, something that you can control and live with, quite happily. It isn't a death sentence – it isn't even an 'illness sentence'. It is simply something that you have found out about yourself that you can cope with. It doesn't make you a different person from the one you were before you were told about it. This book will help you put it in perspective and get on with your life.

6

Managing your blood pressure

Why treat high blood pressure at all? This is a perfectly reasonable question, especially if, when you didn't know you had it, you felt perfectly well. And then you didn't feel so well once you started treatment? That's the case for many people recently given the diagnosis of CKD who are found, incidentally, also to have high blood pressure.

Doctors are always hearing four arguments against treating high blood pressure. They are:

1 I felt well when I had the high blood pressure, but the drugs you give me have unpleasant side effects. Why should I take a drug that makes me feel worse?
2 I've heard that lots of people with high blood pressure live normally into old age with no problems, when the statistics suggest that they should have died years before. Why couldn't I be in that group?
3 You can't prove to me that, as an individual, using drugs to keep my blood pressure low will prolong my life. So why should I take them?
4 Treating high blood pressure involves me not only taking drugs but also changing almost all aspects of my life. Is the change worth the bother?

The best way for us to answer these questions is to tell you about the risks you run if we don't control your blood pressure. There are two kinds of evidence for these risks:

- what happens to people with hypertension as they grow older; and
- the statistics for deaths from hypertension, including from life assurance companies, which base their premium rates on blood pressure measurements – their figures are carefully calculated,

and they are the most accurate measure of the extent to which hypertension shortens life.

However, my feelings on hypertension as a doctor are based on my experiences with patients in the days before we had really effective treatments for it. In my medical student days there were always patients suffering from the last stages of high blood pressure, many of them still young. Two of them I still remember well. One was a schoolteacher, aged 40, with a loving family and everything to live for, who died of a heart attack after a series of strokes. The other was a young woman who developed severe hypertension in her first pregnancy and 2 years later died of kidney failure.

Today, neither would have died. The schoolteacher would have responded well to today's drugs and would have expected to live into a normal old age. The young mother would have had her pregnancy high blood pressure managed efficiently and would not have gone on into kidney failure. However, until the 1970s, high blood pressure often ended up as a condition called malignant hypertension with the sufferer going blind, suffering minor strokes, and dying from kidney failure because of the damage the extreme pressure did to the delicate circulation in his or her nephrons. Once you developed malignant hypertension, you didn't survive a year, despite the best of treatment.

Doctors who have qualified since the 1970s have never seen a full-blown case of malignant hypertension, purely because we now have powerful and highly effective antihypertensive drugs. We not only know that they work, we also know how they work and on which part of the body's pressure-regulating system they act. This is a huge advantage, especially for high blood pressure linked to kidney disease.

This, for me, is the best argument for active treatment of all cases of hypertension – even when it is classified as 'moderate' or 'mild'. You may find it inconvenient, but it is far better than the alternative.

How high blood pressure harms you

Just to hammer an extra nail in the coffin of untreated high blood pressure, and for you to read when you think you might stop your treatment, I outline here the ways in which your circulation reacts to untreated high blood pressure.

The arteries

Your blood vessels take the brunt of the constantly high pressure, and they have to change to cope with it. Their walls thicken to withstand the extra force applied to them. Their inner linings, normally smooth to allow fast flow of the blood inside them, become roughened, so that the diameter of the channel through which the blood has to flow narrows.

In these narrowed, roughened, thickened arteries the blood flow becomes sluggish. The blood becomes stickier as it is pushed by the pressure through the narrowed vessels, and it tends to clot more easily than usual. The scene is set for a thrombosis – in thrombosis, a lump of solid clotted blood, attached to the roughened artery wall, closes the artery off completely. If it is in a coronary artery, which supplies the heart, you will have a heart attack. If it is in a cerebral artery, which supplies the brain, you will have a stroke.

Alternatively, the high pressure may rupture a weakened artery in the brain so that blood escapes into the brain substance. This is a cerebral haemorrhage and leaves you with a severe stroke, with serious after-effects, such as paralysis and loss of feeling; it may be fatal.

The heart

Your heart, too, can be damaged by longstanding untreated high blood pressure. In the beginning the heart copes with the strain of maintaining the high pressure by increasing its muscle bulk, enlarging so that it can pump harder. Eventually it can't enlarge more without losing efficiency. The continuing high pressure expands and thins it, so that it becomes like an overblown balloon.

At this stage the pump starts to fail. The heart can no longer drive the volume of fluid in the circulation around the body, and some of the fluid begins to accumulate in tissues such as the legs and the lungs. The main symptoms are breathlessness on the least exertion and swollen feet and ankles. If the swelling in the feet and ankles is pressed with a finger, a small pit-like depression is left in the waterlogged flesh.

This is congestive heart failure, also known as congestive cardiac failure. In the past it was part of the final weeks of people with CKD. Happily, it is not so today.

The kidneys

I've gone into the mechanisms by which high blood pressure relates to the kidneys in previous chapters, but it is worth reviewing them again. Constant high blood pressure causes the small arteries in the kidneys, including the crucial ones in the glomeruli, to thicken, in exactly the same reaction as the arteries in the heart and brain. It is especially serious for the kidneys, as the result is not simply a matter of poor circulation. The effect is to make the damaged glomeruli less able to perform their function of filtering the blood and producing urine, and to make the tubules less able to restore the correct fluid and electrolyte balance. Hypertensive kidneys will leak more protein and blood into the urine than kidneys of people with normal blood pressure, regardless of whether or not there is also CKD. So it is particularly vital for people with CKD to keep their blood pressure as low as is possible.

In the past, when we didn't have effective antihypertensive drugs, we couldn't tell, when dealing with people in the last stages of kidney failure, whether the initial illness had been kidney disease that had produced high blood pressure or whether it had been high blood pressure that had produced kidney disease. The final clinical pictures of these two situations were identical. It is many years, happily, since a patient in the practices in which I work today has had such uncontrollable hypertension that it led to kidney failure. This is a huge credit to the benefits of modern drugs and to the way today's doctors manage all patients with high blood pressure, regardless of its origin. It is also a credit to the patients whom we treat and who co-operate in such a willing way with our advice.

Evidence for the benefits of treating high blood pressure

The proof that lowering blood pressure into the normal range saves lives – the answer to comment number 3 at the beginning of this chapter – came as long ago as 1982, with the results of two massive trials in Australia and the USA. These trials followed more than

10,000 mildly hypertensive men and women in the two countries. The Australians divided 3,420 subjects, all with only mildly raised blood pressure, into two groups of equal numbers. One group was given active drugs to bring blood pressures into the normal range, the other was given placebo. Over the following 5 years there were four deaths in the 'active' group and 13 in the placebo group – a difference that could not have been expected by chance. Many more people in the placebo group than in the active group also had non-fatal heart attacks and strokes. As the active group had on average a diastolic blood pressure around 5–7mmHg lower than that in the placebo group, it was reasonable to conclude that the lower pressure was the direct cause of the lower death and illness rates.

In the US trial, half of the 7,800 patients were treated intensively by the research doctors themselves, and half were referred back to their GPs for routine blood pressure follow-up. In the 5 years that followed, the 'research' group had significantly lower blood pressures, and 20 per cent fewer deaths, than the GP group. Most of the extra deaths among the GP group were from heart attacks and strokes: only about half of these patients had actually been given antihypertensive drugs.

The doctors who conducted both these studies concluded that mild hypertension should be treated as actively as possible. They made several extra points, too. Professor Austin Doyle, of Melbourne, stressed the importance of treating mild hypertension before it damaged 'end-organs' such as the heart, brain and kidneys. The second point was that most of the patients on placebo in the Australian trial did have satisfactory falls in their blood pressures. He put this down to the better care they were receiving by just being on the trial and from being aware that they needed to do something themselves to improve their blood pressures. They had made personal efforts to do things such as losing excess weight, cutting down on salt, stopping smoking, exercising more and relaxing more.

The big difference in illness and deaths between the two groups of patients came when the diastolic pressures fell below 90, however. Such a fall was rare on placebo alone.

Dr Herbert Langford, of the University of Mississippi, who reported the US results, stressed that the differences in the deaths and illnesses could be explained largely on the finding that those receiving the extra care were known to have stuck more closely to their doctors' instruction and to have taken their drugs more regularly.

Strikingly, among all of the 10,000 patients in the two trials, not one death or serious illness was attributable to a side effect of a drug. So not only were the drugs effective, they were also safer than expected. Minor side effects were reported but no more than on any long-term drug treatment, and very few more than those reported on placebo.

The Americans had not expected such a large drop in deaths in merely 5 years. Spread nationwide, such a saving would prevent tens of thousands of deaths each year. The Australians calculated that in their population of 12 million at the time, if all cases of mild hypertension were treated, there would be 7,000 fewer cases of stroke, heart attack and renal failure, and 2,000 fewer deaths each year. These figures would translate to 9,000 fewer deaths in Britain.

There have been hundreds of studies of antihypertensive treatments since 1982. Probably the two most important, which finally led to worldwide acceptance of the importance of lowering blood pressure, were published in the *Lancet* on 31 March and 7 April 1990. These papers reported the work of doctors in the UK, New Zealand and the USA on 42,000 adults with high blood pressure, followed for between 6 and 25 years.

The first one, on 5,000 patients, showed that reducing the diastolic pressure by only 5mmHg lowered rates of stroke by 34 per cent and heart attack rate by 21 per cent. The corresponding figures for a 10mmHg fall were 56 per cent for stroke and 37 per cent for heart attack.

The second report, written by the same group of doctors, but this time giving the data for 37,000 patients, showed that the protection against stroke and heart attack became significant within 2 years of starting treatment, strokes being reduced by 42 per cent and heart attacks by 14 per cent. In the longer term, the stroke risk continued to be cut by around 40 per cent and the fall in heart attack rates stabilized at around 20–25 per cent.

Since these reports, which have been confirmed again and again as newer drugs have been put to the test, all doctors routinely screen their patients for early rises in blood pressure, and are meticulous in making sure that whenever hypertension is diagnosed, no matter how mild, it is managed correctly. Even when the blood pressure is only marginally raised, in people without CKD, each drop of 2 per cent in average pressure is linked to a 5 per cent drop in risk of a heart attack or stroke. As CKD patients are at higher than average risk in the first place, this is something well worth achieving.

Management of hypertension

So how should we go about treating hypertension, especially in someone with CKD, who is at extra risk of serious illness if his or her blood pressure has started to rise?

The first priority, all the experts agree, is not medication. Everyone with high blood pressure will improve to some extent by changing his or her lifestyle. Some will even improve so much that they will not need drugs. Sadly, this is less likely to be the case for you if you have CKD. It is usually very difficult, as the Australians found, to bring the diastolic pressure below 90mmHg without drugs. It is especially so if you have kidney damage. So don't be surprised if your doctor insists on you taking daily antihypertensive drugs even if your blood pressure is not particularly high.

The next few chapters deal with the non-drug actions you can take to lower your blood pressure – such as controlling cholesterol levels, stopping smoking and taking the appropriate exercise – but first I need to describe the blood pressure-lowering drugs we would choose for you as a CKD patient. They are not necessarily the same as those given to others with hypertension.

7

Drugs to lower blood pressure

This chapter is about drugs that control high blood pressure, but it isn't a catalogue for choosing your own treatment. Of course, today the doctor–patient relationship is a partnership. The old 'doctor knows best' attitude has gone, but decisions on what to prescribe must still be based on good evidence, and your doctor, who works with the British Hypertension Society guidelines, has access to that evidence. So be guided by what your doctor says is best for you as an individual with high blood pressure and CKD. Of course, you can have your input on the decision to prescribe, especially if you feel uncomfortable or have side effects with a particular drug or combination of drugs.

Normal blood pressure is maintained by the co-ordination of different bodily physical and chemical systems. When the blood pressure is too high, that co-ordination has been lost. The different classes of drugs to restore normal blood pressure act on these different systems: how they do so and why they are used is explained here for each type of drug.

The list (in 2008) comprises:

- diuretics
- beta-blockers
- ACE inhibitors
- AT2 blockers
- calcium-channel blockers
- alpha-blockers
- centrally acting agents
- vasodilators
- others best classed as 'miscellaneous'.

The guidelines are straightforward if you have impaired kidney function – an eGFR below 60. In that case, if your systolic pressure is 140mmHg or above or your diastolic pressure is 90 mmHg or above (or both), you should have drug treatment to lower your blood pressure. The choice of drug depends on your particular circumstances.

Initial management

We usually start with a single drug for a week or two, then add another drug in combination treatment if it hasn't brought the pressure down to the target level. If over the next few weeks the combined treatment doesn't control the pressure, then the regimen is re-thought. Your drugs may be replaced by a new combination, or your initial drug doses may be increased, or a new drug is added.

Do accept that finding that you have high blood pressure is hardly ever an emergency. It can take weeks to control. So don't worry if your blood pressure is not quickly brought into the normal range.

There are a few exceptions to this rule. In a very few people, severe high blood pressure causes symptoms (like dizziness, loss of vision, weakness of one side, severe headaches or chest pains), and this indicates that they may soon become ill. In their case, emergency admission to hospital is arranged and appropriate measures taken to bring it down. Our GP guidelines advise that we start treatment immediately if the systolic pressure is at 220mmHg or above or the diastolic is at or above 120mmHg. We have more leeway when the initial levels are lower, but the presence of CKD (with an eGFR below 60 or proteinuria) makes the need for lowering the blood pressure more urgent.

If you find that you don't feel as well as you should after starting on your antihypertensive drug, report it to your doctor. The 'off-feeling' may be a side effect of your drug, and it can often be managed by dropping the dose for a while or changing to another drug or combination.

Keep taking the pills!

You may be tempted to stop the treatment because you feel better without the pills. That is understandable if your blood pressure hasn't made you feel ill in the first place and the treatment has side effects. A diuretic, for example, may make you 'run to the toilet' every few hours, and that can be socially inconvenient. Or a beta-blocker may make you wheeze. Or an ACE inhibitor may cause a cough. But don't succumb to the temptation to stop them without first talking to your doctor. You must learn either to tolerate the side effects or to re-organize your drugs so that the side effects are minimized or abolished. That can mean something as simple as changing the time of day you take the drugs or changing their relationship with meals, or it may mean lowering the dose or changing the drugs. Do what you can to ease the side effect without risking a rise in blood pressure, which is almost inevitable if you stop the tablets.

If you don't take your medicines regularly as advised, your blood pressure will not be under full control. If you don't keep your appointments to have your blood pressure checked, another common failing, you won't know whether the drugs are working to their best effect. Depend on it that your blood pressure will not tell you that it is rising. You may feel better than you did, but have a much higher blood pressure and be heading for a stroke, so don't take the risk. Accept that you have to control your blood pressure for the rest of your life, both to prevent your CKD from worsening and to avoid a heart attack or stroke.

If you do tend to forget to take your pills despite your best intentions, turn them into a daily routine, like brushing your teeth or setting your bedside alarm. Wear a watch with a 12-hour or once-a-day alarm to remind you of your pill times, wherever you are and whatever you are doing.

As insurance, keep a note in your wallet or handbag stating that you have CKD and high blood pressure and giving the details of your medications. Better still, wear a MedicAlert metal disc round your wrist giving the same information. That can save your life in an accident, especially if you need intensive care or surgery. Your surgeon and anaesthetist need to know the drugs that you are taking so that they know what they can and can't give you.

The introduction in the last few years of easy-to-use blood pressure-measuring machines (sphygmomanometers) has helped many people with CKD to follow their blood pressure at home. They find that readings taken a few times a week keep them confident that their treatment is working or can detect an early rise that needs to be discussed with their medical team. I must say here that I have found that some of the new 'sphygmos' give erratic readings that don't correlate with our standard machines in the surgery. So if you are thinking of buying one, please check its accuracy with your doctor's or nurse's sphygmomanometer, to make sure it is accurate. You should choose one that employs a cuff around the upper arm.

Diuretics

Diuretics work by making the kidneys expel more fluid and salt than usual. This shrinks the volume of blood that the heart has to pump around the body, giving it less work to do. The lower blood sodium level (ordinary salt is in fact sodium chloride) causes the walls of the small arteries to relax, thereby opening them up so that the blood can flow through them faster and more smoothly, and reducing the resistance that the heart has to pump against. So diuretics lower both the systolic pressure (the heart's pump pressure) and the diastolic pressure (the tension in the small arteries). They are normally given in low doses because raising their dose if they don't work satisfactorily does not increase their effect, but it does increase their side effects. In CKD, sadly, diuretics don't often work as well as they do in people without kidney disease, and a special type, a 'loop' diuretic that works mainly on the tubules, may have to be given in high dosage.

Their side effects can be troublesome. Apart from having to pass urine more often, high doses of diuretics have been linked with gout, kidney stones, impotence, rashes, fatigue and even increased sensitivity to light. In very high doses they can induce a pre-diabetic state in susceptible people, and they can raise cholesterol level, so that in trials they have been shown to raise the risk of heart attacks. These trials led to guidelines to doctors to keep doses low – and not to raise them if they don't have the desired effect. That is often the case in CKD.

People taking diuretics must have regular blood tests to measure kidney function and their levels of electrolytes (sodium, chloride and potassium). The key electrolyte for CKD patients is potassium, since some diuretics cause it to be excreted along with sodium: if potassium levels drop too low you are put at risk of abnormal heart rhythms. A potassium supplement may have to be given to avoid this, or you may be prescribed a potassium-sparing diuretic.

Diuretics are divided into thiazides and loop diuretics. Thiazides are generally the ones used for uncomplicated hypertension. Loop diuretics have a more severe action and tend to be reserved for conditions in which getting rid of excess fluid is a priority, such as in CKD or heart failure. More than one diuretic may be given together for added effect.

Thiazides include:

- bendroflumethiazide
- cyclopenthiazide
- hydrochlorothiazide
- hydroflumethiazide
- polythiazide.

Thiazide-like diuretics include:

- chlortalidone
- metolazone
- xipamide.

Potassium-sparing diuretics include:

- amiloride
- spironolactone
- triamterene.

Loop diuretics include:

- bumetanide
- ethacrynic acid
- furosemide
- torasemide.

Diuretics that do not fit exactly into the above categories, but that are also used for high blood pressure, are indapamide and metyrapone.

Beta-blockers

Beta-blockers act by slowing and reducing the force of the heartbeat. They can also prevent or correct abnormal heart rhythms. They reduce the systolic pressure rather than the diastolic pressure. They are not all the same. They used to be divided into first-, second- and third-generation drugs, which differ in the details of their actions and side effects, but the division is less clear-cut than was thought. Today there are so many beta-blockers that even doctors who prescribe them every day can be confused by the claims made for them. I have tried here to simplify them, but I will understand if you skip the following paragraphs!

First-generation beta-blockers

First-generation beta-blockers, such as propranolol and oxprenolol, are effective in lowering blood pressure, but they may cause narrowing of the small arteries in the limbs, so that they make the toes and fingers feel cold. This narrowing is emphatically not what we want in the small arteries of the kidneys in people with CKD, so they are rarely the drugs of first choice for you. They may also make you wheeze, worsening any asthma that you may have, and by keeping the heart rate slow, they make it more difficult for you to exercise to the full. They also tend to push up the blood level of the 'wrong' cholesterol – low-density lipoprotein cholesterol – which promotes the deposit of fats in the walls of small arteries, also not an effect you need if you have CKD. Finally, they can also raise blood glucose levels, so if you have CKD and diabetes this is bad news.

Therefore, the initial, first-generation beta-blockers are rarely chosen today as a first-line or even a second-line treatment for high blood pressure in CKD.

Newer beta-blockers

The effects of second-generation beta-blockers (such as atenolol, bisoprolol, metoprolol and nadolol) are more concentrated on the heart than on other sites, so they are less likely to give you cold extremities. And they have less effect on cholesterol. However, they share the 'wheeze' effect with the first-generation drugs.

Third-generation beta-blockers (such as celiprolol and nebivolol) have the advantage of opening up, rather than closing down, the small arteries, so they definitely don't cause cold extremities. Nor do they change cholesterol levels for the worse. They have less effect, too on the lungs.

There are also 'cardioselective' beta-blockers (such as acebutolol, betaxolol, indoramin, oxprenolol and pindolol) that are even less likely to cause cold extremities and wheeze, and that allow you to exercise more; and combined receptor blockers (such as carvedilol and labetalol), which have no effect on the skin or on blood cholesterol.

It is obvious from these lists of side effects that standard beta-blockers are not the drugs of choice for many people, including people with asthma, diabetes or CKD. If you have been prescribed one of them for your hypertension, do discuss it with your doctor, to see if it is correct for you.

ACE inhibitors

ACE inhibitors work by blocking the formation of angiotensin-2. The action of angiotensin-2 is described in Chapter 2, but it bears repeating here, for it is vital to understanding why you may have been prescribed them.

The kidney produces renin when it gets the signal that its circulation is in distress: the blood flow through the glomeruli may be too poor so that they lack oxygen; the aim of the response is to raise the pressure of blood flow through it. Renin is secreted into the circulation from the kidney cells, and this produces a series of chemical reactions that lead to the formation, ultimately, of angiotensin-2. This chemical narrows the small arteries throughout the body, promoting a more powerful heartbeat and higher systolic and diastolic pressures.

Unfortunately, the reaction doesn't help the ailing kidney, because its arteries narrow too, leading to a vicious circle. With the higher pressure, the circulation through the kidneys, already compromised, becomes even poorer, and more renin is formed. This results in even higher blood pressure, and more damage. Inevitably, people with CKD, because of their excessive renin output, produce high levels of angiotensin-2, and their blood pressures remain at very high levels.

ACE inhibitors, which block the final pathway into angiotensin-2, directly stop the vicious circle and initiate the reverse situation. Angiotensin-2 levels fall, and the blood pressure falls accordingly. Better still, there is a direct effect on the circulation within the kidneys, opening up the glomerular arteries and improving their filtration capacity. So ACE inhibitors help not only to reduce the blood pressure, a good end in itself, but also improve the state of the kidneys.

ACE inhibitors have other beneficial effects for people with CKD. They suppress the effects of the hormone aldosterone, which causes the kidneys to retain salt in the circulation. I've already explained that retaining salt pushes up the pressure by increasing the total volume of blood in the circulation. Blocking it has the same effect as reducing salt intake in food.

Unlike beta-blockers, ACE inhibitors can be used in people with heart failure, asthma or diabetes, and in people with longstanding lung disease and poor circulation in the limbs. However, they still have their problems. Many people who start to take them find they have a troublesome cough that is difficult to shift. Some people find that they can no longer taste food as well as before. They may cause rashes, and they can't be used in pregnancy.

The first dose of an ACE inhibitor may cause such a steep drop in blood pressure that it causes you to faint, so it is usually started at a low dose that is gradually increased. This is particularly true if you are already taking a diuretic.

There is one serious problem with ACE inhibitors in CKD. If you have a particular form of fixed narrowing of the arteries leading to the kidneys – the medical term for this is renal artery stenosis – then ACE inhibitors can cause a virtual collapse of the blood supply to the kidneys. The glomeruli can't perform their task, and you can be precipitated into serious renal failure. So if there is any suspicion that you have renal artery stenosis you won't be offered an ACE inhibitor as treatment until it has been ruled out. Most renal artery stenosis is detected after your first visit to the nephrologist or urologist, so you should know whether or not you have it. However, to be certain, if you already have known circulation problems in your limbs, or you have coronary artery disease, you are at higher than normal risk of a renal artery stenosis. You will therefore be investigated fully for it before being given an ACE inhibitor.

As an extra precaution, after starting ACE inhibitors in people with CKD, we watch the blood electrolytes and the progress of the eGFR for the next few weeks and months. If the eGFR starts to fall, the prescription is reconsidered. ACE inhibitors also tend to raise blood potassium levels, so they should not be given with potassium-sparing diuretics or with potassium supplements. Working as a locum in 2007, in a practice in which two doctors had sadly been ill and in which patients had seen several different locums over the previous few months, I was asked to see a woman who felt generally very unwell. She had an abnormal heart rhythm, and it was only when we discovered that she had been taking a high dose of an ACE inhibitor along with the potassium-sparing diuretic amiloride that we realized what was wrong. Her blood potassium level was well above the upper limit of normal, and her heart was reacting badly to it. Once the diuretic was stopped and the dose of ACE inhibitor reduced, she began to feel much better. Happily she came to no permanent harm, and her heart is now normal again.

I must add here a final comment on ACE inhibitors that we cannot explain. If you are of Afro-Caribbean background you may respond less well to ACE inhibitors than people of European background do, and to achieve their full effect you may also need an added diuretic – provided it is not a potassium-sparing one.

ACE inhibitors are easily recognized, since their names all end in -pril. They include:

- captopril
- cilazapril
- enalapril
- fosinopril
- imidapril
- lisinopril
- moexipril
- perindopril
- quinapril
- ramipril
- transolapril.

Which one your doctor chooses depends as much on his or her experience with the drug as on its relative merits from clinical trials.

AT2 blockers

AT2 blockers work in a similar way to ACE inhibitors, in that they stop angiotensin-2 from increasing blood pressure. Their advantage is that they don't cause the dry cough that so often bothers ACE inhibitor users. In my experience in general practice, about one in five people on ACE inhibitors have had to change to AT2 blockers. This seems a higher proportion than we read about in the journals, a higher proportion that I can't explain. The names of all the AT2 blockers end in –sartan. They include:

- candesartan
- irbesartan
- losartan
- valsartan.

Calcium-channel blockers

For a muscle cell to contract, it needs free calcium ions (electrically charged calcium molecules) inside it. Calcium-channel blockers block the channels in the walls of muscle cells that allow calcium to enter them from the tissue fluid around them. They also prevent the release of calcium ions from stores within the cells.

When the smooth muscle cells in the walls of arteries are low in free calcium ions, they cannot contract fully. Their more relaxed state opens up the arteries around which they are placed, lowering the resistance to flow of blood within them. The blood pressure therefore falls. The heart muscle is affected in the same way when calcium entry into it is blocked, so that the strength of the heart-beat diminishes. Therefore, both the systolic and diastolic pressures fall.

Calcium-channel blockers, or calcium antagonists, differ in their details. They are usually defined as ether 'dihydropyridines' or 'others'. The dihydropyridines are normally used for hypertension alone, and the others are also used for problems with heart rhythms and for some types of heart failure.

Dihydropyridines can be recognized because their names all end in -ipine. They include:

- amlodipine
- felodipine
- israpidine
- lacidipine
- lercanidipine
- nicardipine
- nifedipine
- nisoldipine.

The 'others' include diltiazem and verapamil.

Calcium-channel blockers have no effect on blood lipids, blood glucose or angiotensin-2. They do not cause retention of salt and they do not stimulate gout. They have no effect on the lungs. They are useful in older people, in people of Afro-Caribbean background (who may not respond so well to beta-blockers or diuretics) and in people with asthma, diabetes, kidney disease and poor circulation in the legs and feet.

Past preparations of calcium-channel blockers caused headaches, flushing, palpitations and ankle swelling. With today's preparations, in which the effect of one tablet is stretched out over 24 hours, these side effects have become much less common. If you are taking one of these newer 'sustained-release' calcium-channel blockers, make sure you are dispensed the same brand with each repeat prescription, because different preparations of the same drug may have different effects on your circulation throughout the day and night. Calcium-channel blockers are often given along with beta-blockers if the beta-blocker has caused cold fingers and toes.

Alpha-blockers

Alpha-blockers lower blood pressure by blocking the activity of the nerves that control the muscles that cause the small arteries to narrow. Under alpha-blockade these small arteries open up, so that the diastolic pressure can fall steeply after the first dose. This fall can be dramatic, so alpha-blockers may have the effect of 'first-dose fainting', especially if you stand up quickly from a sitting or lying position. You can minimize this risk by starting on a low dose and stopping any diuretic treatment beforehand.

Because of these side effects alpha-blockers are not usually given to older people who may already have problems with dizziness on standing. Other side effects of alpha-blockers include tiredness, weakness, a stuffy nose and headache.

On the positive side, alpha-blockers reduce total cholesterol levels while increasing the 'good' HDL cholesterol, so that they are recommended in some people known to have heart disease or diabetes, and in some cases of CKD. Alpha-blockers are also helpful in reducing the volume of a benignly enlarged prostate.

Alpha-blockers include:

- doxazosin
- indoramin
- prazosin
- terazosin.

Centrally acting drugs and vasodilators

A full review of the drugs prescribed to reduce high blood pressure in the UK today wouldn't be complete without at least a mention of centrally acting and vasodilator drugs. You are unlikely to be prescribed them unless you have had extraordinary difficulty in establishing control of your blood pressure using the standard drugs described above.

Centrally acting drugs

The three centrally acting drugs are moxonidine, clonidine and methyldopa. They all work on the centre within the brain that controls the nerve signals sent to the muscles around the small arteries. By lessening the signals, these drugs cause the tone in the muscles to decrease, and the arteries open up, with the usual results. Methyldopa is a very old drug, dating from the 1950s, and we know its effects and side effects very well. The most common is woolly-headedness, but its main problem is that the dose often has to be raised every few weeks as the brain begins to 'tolerate' effects of the drug. A major problem with moxonidine and clonidine is that you can get a 'rebound' steep increase in blood pressure if they are stopped suddenly, with possibly disastrous results. Methyldopa was abandoned in most practices years ago, and I don't know of any CKD patient in the practices in which I am a regular locum who is taking either moxonidine or clonidine for his or her blood pressure.

Vasodilators

Vasodilators open up the small arteries by a direct action on the muscles in the artery walls. They include:

- hydralazine
- diazoxide
- minoxidil.

They tend to be used when there have been difficulties such as side effects or lack of effect with the mainstream drugs. Their side effects include gut disturbances, such as indigestion, bloating and wind, and fluid retention, with swollen ankles. Minoxidil in particular is used in people whose blood pressure has not responded to beta-blockers or diuretics. Its ability to produce unwanted hair growth has led to its other use. When rubbed into a bald scalp as an ointment (the trade name for this preparation of the drug is Regaine) it can stimulate new hair growth.

To summarize this chapter

This chapter looks at the different drug choices your GP and consultant have to make when considering the best way for you to reduce your blood pressure. Armed with this information, you should now be able to understand why your particular choice was made for you. The aim is to protect the delicate tissues of your arteries, throughout your body but particularly in your kidneys, from the effects of higher than normal blood pressure.

However, your arteries need protection, too, from another coronary- and stroke-producing menace, cholesterol. As most people with CKD that has been diagnosed from a chance eGFR test result also have atheroma (see Chapter 2) you will almost certainly have been advised to lower your cholesterol levels, too. The next chapter explains why it is so important.

8

Your cholesterol risk

To understand the role of blood lipids like cholesterol in protecting our circulation and our kidneys, we need to know more about the 'good' and 'bad' lipids, how they come to be in the blood at all, and what they do.

Why do we need cholesterol, considering that it does so much damage to our arteries? I can best answer that by posing a *Trivial Pursuit*-type question. What is the fattest organ in the body – the one that contains the highest proportion of fat in comparison with protein or glucose? The answer is the brain.

The brain needs a lot of fat, because fat is an essential component of nerve cells and their insulating covering, a substance called myelin. Without myelin separating nerve cell fibres from each other, the electrical signal that runs along the fibres would dissipate into the surrounding tissues, and the nervous system would not work. This is, in fact, the problem in people with multiple sclerosis: their myelin sheaths deteriorate, and their nerves fail to work.

So we need to transport fats around our bodies to keep our organs healthy and working to maximum capacity. We do that by using the 'family' of fats, one group of which is cholesterol-based.

Cholesterol has a complex chemical structure, the details of which are outside the remit of this book. Its building blocks are derived from fatty acids that we obtain, in the first place, from fats in our food. The story goes like this. We swallow food containing fat or oil. They are digested into fatty acids, and pass to the liver, which turns them into cholesterol. This passes into the bloodstream, where it is transported into the tissues that need it, and it is converted into the type of fat needed by the organ. For example, it can be myelin for nervous tissue; or phospholipids (fats attached to phosphate molecules) or lipoproteins (fats combined with proteins) for specialist jobs in brain and nerve cells; for fat in breast milk; or simpler fats for storage around our gut or under the skin.

Fat storage is a relic from our hundreds of thousands of years as hunter–gatherers, when we had to face many times of near-famine. We ate as much as we could in times of plenty so that we could live on our fat stores in times of near-starvation. Conversely, our usual immediate source of energy is glucose, which we make in our gut from the digestion of sugars and starches, but we have very limited capacity to store it. In fact glucose is stored as a substance called glycogen in some muscles and the liver, but all our body's supply of glycogen can quickly be used up when we exert ourselves. From then on we have to use stored fats as our energy source.

We inherited from our Stone Age ancestors a very efficient system for storing fats, so that they can be used as fuel for our muscles, brain and other organs when we have nothing to eat or have used up our glucose and glycogen. Conditions 10,000 or more years ago probably kept our ancestors thin, so that they used up all the fat they could consume in their daily lives. Today, everyone in developed societies has enough to eat. If we do not use up all the fat and glucose we eat each day in energetic activity, then we have to store it, and almost all of it is stored as fat. Even among people with a normal body shape who are not obese, the average woman is 18 per cent fat, and the average man is 10 per cent fat.

However, fewer and fewer of us have normal body shapes. We exercise far less than we used to, and we eat and drink more. Today, by the time we reach 50 years of age, nearly half of us, men and women, are overweight enough to be described as obese. Obese people are at least 30 per cent fat, and perhaps a lot more.

Where does that fat go, and what does it consist of? We may put it on our waists, our hips or our backs (in a 'buffalo hump'), or we may space it fairly equally under the skin all round our torso and limbs. It is also laid down in the walls of our arteries, as streaks and plaques. Classically, people are described as 'apples' (with fat mainly around the waist and inside the abdomen) or 'pears' (with most of the fat around the hips and bottom). There is some evidence that apples are more prone to heart attacks than pears, because they lay down more fat in their artery walls than the pears do, but any form of obesity raises the risks.

However, the message of this chapter isn't just about obesity. There are some (not many) obese people with relatively low levels of 'bad' cholesterol in their blood, and there are thin people (again, not many) who have high levels of 'bad' cholesterol. And of the two, those with the high cholesterol levels, whether they are fat or thin, are more likely to have a heart attack or stroke.

This, then, is where we must explain about 'bad' and 'good' cholesterol. The medical name for fat of any sort is lipid. Blood lipid level is the term for the amount of fats in your venous blood, taken usually from a vein in your arm. The lipids we are most concerned about fall into two main categories, cholesterol and triglyceride. However, the lipids don't float about in the blood on their own. Most molecules of cholesterol and triglyceride in the blood are transported around attached to proteins, so they are called lipoprotein complexes. We identify the different types of lipoprotein complex by spinning the plasma (blood from which the red cells have been removed) in a centrifuge. That separates out the different lipoproteins from each other according to how dense (heavy) they are.

There are:

- very low-density lipoproteins (VLDLs)
- low-density lipoproteins (LDLs)
- high-density lipoproteins (HDLs).

Triglyceride is usually carried in VLDLs, and cholesterol is usually carried in LDLs or HDLs. In your blood test report, TC means total cholesterol, LDL-C means the LDL-cholesterol level, and similarly for VLDL-C and HDL-C. TG stands for triglyceride level. Don't confuse TC with TG, which means triglycerides.

The body attaches fats to proteins (to form lipoproteins) because this is the only way in which lipids can be transported across the healthy small artery walls. When it is combined with protein, the fat molecule is soluble and is therefore easy for the artery walls to handle. As a free fat in the blood, either as cholesterol or triglyceride, it remains relatively insoluble, cannot cross the intact artery wall and so remains in the blood. However, if the artery wall is damaged, it is a different story. Without an intact layer of healthy artery lining cells to protect the blood vessel wall, the fats and triglyceride can pass into the wall, where they are laid down as solid deposits, helping to form the structure of plaques.

Your blood test result will indicate your levels of triglyceride, HDL-cholesterol and LDL-cholesterol, along with your TC. Local hospital laboratories all over the world measure blood lipid levels in their own populations, and relate the results in each individual to their normal range. The normal range differs from country to country, within areas in the same country, and even within populations in different districts in the same city. So it is difficult to be precise in a book like this on what is 'normal' and what is 'high' for you.

However, specialists in diseases of blood vessels and lipid disorders have defined what they see as acceptable generally for everyone. Everyone with a blood lipid 'profile' that causes concern is given a general diagnosis of 'dyslipidaemia'. The term simply means abnormal levels of fat in the blood. If you have a higher than normal level of TC or LDL-cholesterol this is called hypercholesterolaemia (from *hyper* meaning 'too much'; cholesterol; and *aemia* meaning 'in the blood'). Too high a triglyceride level is called hypertriglyceridaemia, and when both cholesterol and triglyceride are raised, it is called combined hyperlipidaemia.

Some people have low HDL-cholesterol levels, but their other lipids are in the normal range: they are diagnosed as having dyslipidaemia. However, a low HDL-cholesterol almost always goes with hypertriglyceridaemia, so low HDL-cholesterol on its own is relatively rare.

All of these types of dyslipidaemia may be inborn (inherited with your genes) or 'secondary' (brought on by lifestyle), or they can be a combination of both.

Crucial to the recognition of dyslipidaemias is that they are very strongly related to your risk of having heart attacks and strokes. In particular, the worse your hypercholesterolaemia or hypertriglyceridaemia, or both, the higher is your risk of succumbing to one of these catastrophes. The risk rises throughout the range of blood cholesterol, from the lowest of all to the highest, and the slope of the rising risk is a steep one.

We measure lipid levels in the UK in millimoles of each type of lipid per litre (mmol/l) of blood. A man with a TC of 5.2 mmol/l has half the risk of coronary heart disease (angina and heart attack) of a man with a TC of 6.5 mmol/l and only a quarter of the risk of a man with a TC of 7.8mmol/l. Put another way, if you reduce your TC from 7.8 mmol/l to 5.2 mmol/l, you will reduce your heart attack risk to one-quarter of what it was.

This is not guesswork. It has been proved time and time again in populations within countries and in comparisons between countries. Countries with low TC levels, like Japan (average around 4.9mmol/l), have about 60 coronary and stroke deaths per 100,000 people per year; in those with averages above 6 mmol/l, like my own country, Scotland, the corresponding figure is 600. Finland used to have similar figures – 10 times those of Japan – but since its government initiated a huge healthy lifestyle campaign both the TC levels and the numbers of deaths have plummeted. The relationship between TC levels and deaths from heart attacks is constant for almost every country. Take Poland, with a TC average of 5.5 mmol/l and a 'heart' death rate of 280 per 100,000, or Germany with 5.7 mmol/l and 320, and England with 6.5 mmol/l and 470. One 'outlier', or exception, is France with an average TC of 5.8 mmol/l and a death rate of only 135. This lower 'heart' death rate than expected is almost certainly explained by the regular consumption in France of red wine, which seems to protect against deposition of fats in artery walls.

However, a rise in TC alone does not explain all the cholesterol-related deaths. When concerns were raised in the 1950s about the steep increase in heart disease, health experts all over the world started to study their own populations 'prospectively'. That is, they selected healthy people for close follow-up over many years, having first measured their blood lipid profiles. In some trials people were left to follow their usual lifestyles without interference, whereas other trials promoted what was thought then to be a healthier lifestyle for hearts to some subjects, and not to others. The goal was to follow as many of the people as possible to their eventual deaths, and to record their age at death and the cause of death.

The results of most of these studies were published in the 1980s, and they became the basis for almost all we do today about managing high blood lipid levels. Certainly they provided the motivation to doctors to ensure that their patients should keep their lipid profiles as healthy as possible.

All the studies confirmed that men with higher TC levels were more likely to die from heart attacks and strokes than those with lower TC levels. But in each study there were substantial numbers of men with low TC levels who still died early. This was true in countries in continental Europe, the USA and the UK. In the British Regional Heart Study, one in five of the men recorded as having serious or fatal heart attacks or strokes had TCs below 6 mmol/l. They were in the lowest 40 per cent of the range of TC results.

Why did so many people with relatively low TCs die? There are several ways of explaining this. Perhaps a TC of 6 mmol/l is still far too high for safety. It is certainly very much higher than the average Japanese TC. We should probably aim for a TC under 5 mmol/l. Or there may be other aspects of their lipids, such as a high TG and LDL-cholesterol with a low HDL-cholesterol, that were not measured in the studies. Alternatively, other factors, such as high blood pressure, smoking habit or diabetes, may have played their part.

In fact, all of these explanations are true. Why should some lipids, like LDL-cholesterol and TG, be thought to be 'bad' for us, and HDL-cholesterol be thought to be 'good'? Let's go back to the idea of fats being deposited into the blood vessel walls, where they cause plaques of atheroma and eventually block or rupture the artery. How does that happen? The most recent view is as follows.

The liver receives fatty acids, as described above (see p. 70), from the bowel after our digestion has formed them by breaking down fats in our food. The liver cells then start the process of turning the fatty acids into TG and cholesterol. The combination of the two with protein forms VLDL-cholesterol. This is the most suitable form of fat for release from the liver into the bloodstream. Once in the bloodstream, it is then ready for delivery to the smallest blood vessels for transport across the walls of the small arteries into the tissues. On the way, the VLDL-cholesterol is progressively enriched with more cholesterol, which makes the molecules more dense, forming LDL-cholesterol. The artery walls are therefore faced with VLDL-cholesterol and LDL-cholesterol, which they must carry across into the tissues beyond, so that the fat can be used for the building and energy processes described above.

So far, so good. But what happens if there is too much VLDL-cholesterol and LDL-cholesterol? Some of it circulates back to the liver, where it is taken up by the liver cells and stored for future use. Some of it is taken up by fat storage cells. But a sizeable proportion of it remains in the connective tissue layer just beyond the artery walls, where it is treated by the body as an irritant, and 'scavenged' by white blood cells called to the site to deal with it. The white cells fill with cholesterol, and become 'foam' cells, so named because under the microscope they look as if they are filled with foam.

Foam cells do not survive long. They die, releasing free cholesterol into the artery wall. If this state continues, platelets (tiny solid cell remnants that circulate in the blood) are attracted to the area, and form tiny 'thromboses', on the surface. This is the beginning of a plaque. High levels of VLDL-cholesterol (containing mainly triglyceride) and LDL-cholesterol (containing mainly cholesterol) are therefore a recipe for forming and maintaining and enlarging plaques. They are justifiably called 'bad' lipids.

Where does HDL-cholesterol fit into this? The artery wall does try to heal itself and to get rid of the cholesterol and triglyceride gathering like a microscopic blackhead around it. The only way it can do that is to make the LDL-cholesterol and the VLDL-cholesterol even denser. Only by collecting the fats into high-density lipoprotein masses, by turning VLDL-cholesterol and LDL-cholesterol into HDL-cholesterol, can the arteries manage to extrude the fats from the deposits in their walls back into the bloodstream. Once the fat is in the bloodstream, the only organ to take it up in any serious amount is the liver, which can then turn it into bile and excrete it.

So HDL-cholesterol is the body's answer to excessive fat deposits: it is made by the endothelium to protect itself. A high HDL-cholesterol level means that there is a good turnover of lipids in the body, in the direction of lowering fatty deposits in the artery walls. HDL-cholesterol is justifiably the 'good' cholesterol.

How can we bring all these facts about cholesterol and blood lipids together? The first message is that the higher your total cholesterol is, the more likely you are to have a heart attack or stroke, and the more likely you are to have it earlier, rather than later, in your life. The second message is that TC is not the only risk. TC is only a rough guide. Within it are VLDL-cholesterol (mainly trigly-ceride), LDL-cholesterol (mainly cholesterol), and HDL-cholesterol. Raise the first two, and lower the third, and you make a heart attack or stroke more likely. Lower the first two and raise the third, and you reduce your chance of a heart attack or stroke.

Most of today's management of people with high cholesterol is now devoted to lowering TG and LDL-cholesterol and if possible to raising HDL-cholesterol at the same time. How we do that is described in Chapter 10.

Summary

The higher your blood cholesterol level is, the more fat is likely to be deposited in the walls of your arteries, as 'plaques'. The longer it continues to be high the greater number and the bigger the plaques will be. The more plaques in your arteries, the higher is your chance of having a heart attack or stroke, or both. It is as simple as that. Lower your cholesterol level, and you will substantially lower that chance.

This is good sense for anyone, but it is particularly important for you if you have CKD. We know that even mild CKD – with eGFRs around 50 to 60 – is linked to coronary and stroke risks around 25 per cent higher than among people of similar body shape and life-style with no kidney disease.

Obviously you mustn't depend on lowering cholesterol alone. You must also tackle other aspects of your life that harm your arteries. If you have high blood pressure that is not well controlled, then those muscles wrapped round your arteries will grow thicker and narrow your arteries, making a blockage much more likely. It will also put extra strain on areas of plaque, so that they can split asunder, tear the artery wall, and cause a bleed. In the brain that is a haemorrhagic stroke.

If you smoke, then you directly damage your arterial walls with each inhalation you take. The thousand or so damaging chemicals in smoke pass into your blood, and they poison the very delicate single layer of cells that lines every artery. Smokers have very many fewer functioning active artery lining cells than non-smokers. This leads to many problems for the circulation. For a start, they cannot give the signal to the muscle layer to relax, so that the calibre of the tube through which the blood has to flow is greatly reduced. That means less oxygen getting through to the tissues beyond. In fact smoking already compromises the oxygen supply to the artery wall because so many red cells of a smoker carry carbon monoxide, rather than oxygen, around the body. And you can't use carbon monoxide for energy! It is the same deadly poison that used to kill people when they put their heads in gas ovens using the old town gas.

Smoking also harms the arteries by promoting blood clotting. It increases the blood levels of a substance, fibrinogen, that is the most powerful natural blood-clotting agent. It also makes the blood stickier so that elements of it, called platelets, stick to the artery walls and to each other far more easily. Once stuck together they stay stuck. Clots develop on top of heaps of stuck-together platelets.

Then there is nicotine itself. Smokers of even one cigarette a day put enough nicotine in their blood to cause the muscles around the arteries to contract – making the arteries, already under an onslaught, even narrower. If you were deliberately to try to design a drug that would kill people with a heart attack or stroke, you could not possibly do better than tobacco.

Finally, if you have diabetes, constantly higher than normal levels of glucose in your blood, along with high blood pressure, can also damage the arteries. So do follow your strict plan for control of your diabetes and blood pressure.

The message of this chapter, therefore, is to look on your arteries in the same way as you look on your brain, lungs, heart, liver and kidneys. Most of us dread the thought of our brain going in old age, and of ending up with dementia. So we try to stave it off by keeping it active. We know about our lungs, and how smoking affects them. We all know of the messages about a healthy heart – no one could have missed the promotion of healthy eating, such as five portions of fruit and vegetables a day, with oily fish and perhaps red wine thrown in. Every so often a celebrity is shown to have liver disease bad enough to need a transplant because of his excessive drinking (footballer George Best springs to mind). And since you are reading this book, you are obviously concerned about your kidneys. But how many of us know that we need to look after our arteries? Or how important cholesterol and other fats in our blood are to keeping our arteries healthy? Yet keeping our arteries healthy is the key to keeping all the other organs healthy, too, including our kidneys.

9

Lowering cholesterol

Who should be treated, and the evidence for drugs

If you have a raised cholesterol level along with your CKD, you are probably taking a lipid-lowering drug, and you perhaps wonder whether they are doing more harm than good. This is a common problem for people who have few, if any, symptoms of disease, yet who are told they must take drugs for the rest of their life if they are to avoid future illness. They naturally fear that taking a drug for years may have an unexpected damaging side effect. Would it be worth stopping the drug and taking the chance that they won't have the predicted heart attack or stroke?

So this chapter first sets out the recommendations by the European Joint Task Force (a group of distinguished specialists in lipid disorders) on who should have lipid-lowering drugs. It then gives the evidence from trials on why the Task Force came to its decisions, and leaves you to decide on whether the benefits of the drugs outweigh the potential drawbacks.

Who shouldn't and who should be offered drug treatment:

Unless you already have been ill with, or are showing early symptoms of, heart disease, if you have mild or moderate hyper-cholesterolaemia that has started to reverse after changing your lifestyle you do not need drugs.

According to the European Joint Task Force, you do need drug treatment if you:

- are a high risk patient (i.e. someone who already has shown signs of heart or kidney disease);
- have other risk factors, such as high blood pressure;
- are at high risk as a result of special risk factors, such as having high lipoprotein (a) (a specific subtype of lipoprotein) or high fibrinogen levels in your blood (both of which indicate fairly severe risk to your arteries);

- have hypercholesterolaemia that has not responded to changes in lifestyle designed to lower your cholesterol;
- have inherited ('familial') hyperlipidaemia with relatives who died early, because this condition is unlikely to respond to lifestyle changes and carries a high risk of heart attack and stroke; or
- have any severe form of dyslipidaemia, or evidence of coronary disease along with mild or moderate dyslipidaemia – people with CKD often come into this category.

You will gather from these guidelines that almost everyone with a high cholesterol or evidence of artery disease is eligible for drug treatment. The Task Force was convinced by the results of trials of the drugs that they provide much more benefit than they do harm. Below is some of the evidence on which they based that judgement.

The Air Force/Texas Coronary Atherosclerosis Prevention Study

The Air Force/Texas Coronary Atherosclerosis Prevention Study (AFCAPS/TexCAPS) was reported to the American Heart Association in 1997. It followed 6,605 men and women with mildly raised cholesterol levels, but no initial evidence of heart disease, who were given either a statin (in this case, lovastatin) or placebo.

AFCAPS/TexCAPS was stopped early because of the far greater 'event rate' (numbers of people with heart attacks and strokes) among those taking the placebo than in those on the statin. Among those on the statin there were 40 per cent fewer fatal and non-fatal heart attacks, 32 per cent fewer serious attacks of angina and a 33 per cent reduction in the number of people needing emergency coronary artery surgery compared with those taking the placebo. Women, the elderly, smokers, people with high blood pressure and people with diabetes all benefited from the statin, and the improvement was seen even in those with the mildest rise in blood lipid levels.

Atorvastatin Versus Revascularization Treatments

The 341 people who entered the Atorvastatin Versus Revascularization Treatments (AVERT) study all had known coronary artery disease with angina. They had all had angiograms that showed they had narrowing of at least one coronary artery. Then they were allocated randomly to either medical treatment with a statin (atorvastatin) or to angioplasty (in which a balloon-tipped catheter is used to expand the narrowed coronary segment). Angioplasty is regarded as the standard treatment of coronary artery narrowing in people with angina. It is usually highly successful and has been a great addition to our ability to treat people with angina. It is routinely used during heart attacks in specialist hospitals to prevent heart muscle damage.

Of course angioplasties do not guarantee prevention of further attacks of angina or even full heart attacks (in which an artery is completely blocked and the area of heart muscle beyond the blockage dies). Atorvastatin turned out to be more effective than angioplasty. There were 36 per cent fewer new cardiac episodes (attacks of angina or heart attacks) and the time from start of treatment to the next event was longer on the atorvastatin treatment than after the angioplasties. TC, LDL-cholesterol and TG levels were all lower on atorvastatin than after angioplasty. There were fewer serious side effects of treatment on atorvastatin than after angioplasty.

The authors of the AVERT study concluded that atorvastatin may help to postpone angioplasty procedures or even to avoid them completely in some patients with mild or moderate coronary artery disease.

The Cholesterol and Recurrent Events (CARE) study

The Cholesterol and Recurrent Events (CARE) study followed people with high LDL-cholesterol levels who also had already had heart attacks. It enrolled 4,159 patients with TC below 6.2 mmol/l and LDL-cholesterol of 3.0–4.5 mmol/l. These patients would have been borderline candidates for drugs if they had not had a heart attack. Half were given a statin (pravastatin) and half placebo, and they were followed for 5 years. There were 24 per cent fewer heart attacks on pravastatin than on placebo. There were also a 26 per cent less need for coronary artery bypass surgery, a 23 per cent reduction in angioplasty and a 31 per cent reduction in stroke.

Interestingly CARE showed that women responded to pravastatin better than men, with a bigger drop in the rate of heart attack and stroke and a bigger drop in the need for surgery; this was particularly so in women with higher initial LDL-cholesterol values.

The Long-term Intervention with Pravastatin in Ischaemic Disease (LIPID) study

In the 1990s, doctors in 87 centres in Australia and New Zealand entered more than 9,000 patients in a study in which they were given either a statin (pravastatin) or a placebo. All the patients had coronary artery disease and had been previously admitted to hospital because of a heart attack or an attack of severe angina.

The LIPID study had to be stopped early, after 6 years, because of the obvious advantage enjoyed by the statin-treated group. The patients given pravastatin showed reductions of 18 per cent in TC, 25 per cent in LDL-cholesterol and 12 per cent in TG. There was an increase of 6 per cent in HDL-cholesterol. Linked with these changes were reductions of 24 per cent in deaths due to heart events and an overall reduction in deaths from all causes of 22 per cent.

People who were concerned about the costs of prescribing statins to so many patients were reassured by the news that the statin group needed 20 per cent fewer angioplasties and bypass operations. This made the overall costs of drug treatment less than the costs of no drugs with the attendant likely need for patient 'rescue' with extra heart surgery.

The Scandinavian Simvastatin Survival Study

The Scandinavian Simvastatin Survival Study (4S) was one of the earlier studies of the use of statins in people with hypercholesterolaemia. It concentrated on patients with TC levels between 5.5 and 8.0 mmol/l, and for 5 years it followed 4,444 patients allocated to simvastatin or placebo. By the end of the trial there were 34 per cent fewer major heart problems among the patients on simvastatin than among those taking placebo. 4S showed that for each fall of 1 per cent in TC the risk of a major cardiac event fell by 1.9 per cent, and that a 1 per cent fall in LDL-cholesterol led to a reduction of 1.7 per cent in the risk of a major cardiac event.

The West of Scotland Coronary Prevention Study

I must admit bias towards the West of Scotland Coronary Prevention Study (WOSCOPS) because it was conducted in my home area, and I know some of the GPs and the men who took part in it.

WOSCOPS followed 6,595 men who had never had a heart attack, giving them either pravastatin or placebo. Pravastatin certainly worked: there were 36 per cent fewer severe heart events among the patients on it than among those taking placebo. However, this fall could not be related to changes in cholesterol levels from their starting levels or to the cholesterol levels on treatment. The authors of WOSCOPS felt that the benefits of pravastatin were not due to the reduction in LDL-cholesterol alone. They did show that the men with higher than average TG levels (more than 1.6 mmol/l) benefited more from the statin than men with higher than average total cholesterol levels (more than 7 mmol/l), although both groups gained substantial benefit.

The Stockholm Ischaemic Heart Disease Secondary Prevention Study supported this conclusion that lowering TG levels offered considerable benefits. In the patients whose TG was lowered by more than 30 per cent, the deaths from heart disease fell by a massive 60 per cent.

Summary

This chapter could go on and on relating the different trials of drugs in hyperlipidaemia, but enough is enough. The defence of the use of lipid-lowering agents in people with hyperlipidaemias of all types rests. All the trials showed benefit outweighing the risk of adverse events. The current lipid-lowering drugs are described in the next chapter.

10

Drugs to lower cholesterol

Drugs that improve blood lipid levels have been a huge success. The trials described in Chapter 9 are only some among many that have shown that these drugs do what they claim to do – they lower cholesterol and triglyceride levels, and in doing so they prevent deaths from heart attacks and strokes in the people most vulnerable to them.

The best known of these drugs are the statins, although they may not be the correct drugs for everyone with a lipid problem. Today there are four 'lipid-lowering' types of drug:

- statins
- fibrates
- bile-acid sequestrants
- nicotinic acid.

Statins

The statins are also known as hydroxy-methyl-glutaryl coenzyme A (HMG-CoA) reductase inhibitors. Statins in current use include atorvastatin, fluvastatin, pravastatin and simvastatin. They hit the headlines in 2001 when cerivastatin was withdrawn after reports of unacceptably high numbers of cases of muscle pains, especially when given with fibrates.

Statins work by blocking an enzyme, HMG-CoA reductase, which is involved in the making of cholesterol in the liver. They are most effective, therefore, at reducing LDL-cholesterol; they are less effective at lowering high TG levels. Nevertheless they do reduce TG by between 15 and 40 per cent, depending on the dose. Doses range up to 80 mg per day for atorvastatin, fluvastatin and simvastatin, and up to 40 mg per day for pravastatin.

Most people tolerate statins well. The main problem that they can cause is with muscles. A few people given statins develop pains in the muscles, often in the shoulder and upper back. If this happens to you, you should stop the drug and report the effect to your doctor. The muscle problem may be made worse (even to the extent that some of the muscle tissues are destroyed in a process called rhabdomyolysis) if the drug is given with fibrates, which are mainly used to lower TG levels. The problem may also be worsened if you are taking drugs for other illnesses, such as ciclosporin (to prevent transplant rejection), erythromycin (an antibiotic) and ketoconazole (an antifungal drug).

You will not be prescribed statins if you have liver disease or are a heavy drinker, because they can be toxic (poisonous) to a liver that is showing long-term disease such as active hepatitis or alcoholic degeneration of the liver. Your doctor will take blood for liver function tests before you start on a statin and repeat the tests every 6 months.

Other, less often reported side effects include headache, abdominal pain, flatulence, diarrhoea, nausea and vomiting. There have been very rare reports of rashes and allergic reactions to statins. Statins combine well with bile-acid sequestrants, but they must be used with great care with fibrates or nicotinic acid.

By blocking the HMG-CoA reductase enzyme, statins reduce both LDL-cholesterol and VLDL-cholesterol levels, so that they reduce blood TC and TG levels, while slightly increasing HDL-cholesterol. Which statin your doctor chooses to use depends a lot on his or her personal experience with this class of drugs. They are probably all similar in effect and side effects. The statins that are available are unlikely to go the way of cerivastatin.

Fibrates

The fibrates include bezafibrate, ciprofibrate, fenofibrate and gemfibrozil. They lower VLDL-cholesterol by blocking its synthesis in the liver, so that they are useful in treating combined hypercholesterolaemia and hypertriglyceridaemia. They may also stimulate the clearance of excess LDL-cholesterol from the plasma. All fibrates tend to raise HDL-cholesterol, but only by a small amount.

As with the statins, most people have no trouble when they take fibrates. However, there are some reports of nausea, diarrhoea, gallstones, alopecia (hair loss) and muscle weakness with fibrates. Your doctor will wish to monitor the liver regularly, because there are rare cases of liver upsets on fibrates. Very great care must be taken if you are considering taking a fibrate with a statin, as the combination can lead to muscle problems. However, there are few problems in prescribing fibrates along with nicotinic acid or bile-acid sequestrants.

Bile-acid sequestrants

There are two bile-acid sequestrants currently available, cholesty-ramine and colestipol. They work by 'binding' to the bile acids in the gut, so that the bile acids can no longer deliver fats to the liver for processing into new cholesterol and triglyceride. The liver there-fore needs to 'suck' cholesterol back into it from the circulation. This sets up a flow of fats from their deposits in the endothelium through the circulation into the liver. Plasma cholesterol levels therefore fall. However, there may be a downside – VLDL-cholesterol and TG levels may rise.

Cholestyramine and colestipol are used in people with raised LDL-cholesterol, but not in people with hypertriglyceridaemia. They are also not used in people who have constipation. Indeed, constipation is the main side effect of bile-acid sequestrants, and it sometimes proves too inconvenient for people to continue with them, although 'bulking' laxatives usually relieve it.

Bile-acid sequestrants may reduce the absorption of other impor-tant drugs, making them less effective. You should therefore not take them within 3 hours of taking doses of warfarin (which are used to slow blood clotting), thyroxine (thyroid hormone), diuretics and beta-blockers (which are usually given for high blood pressure but sometimes for an abnormal heart rhythm). They may also affect the uptake from the gut of folic acid (given before and during preg-nancy, mainly to prevent spina bifida and other spine and brain abnormalities in developing infants) and vitamins A and D.

People taking bile-acid sequestrants should have their blood monitored for possible malabsorption problems (such as anaemia) each year. They can be given with each of the other lipid-lowering drug types.

Nicotinic acid

Nicotinic acid is a vitamin, but the dose used to lower blood lipid levels is much higher than the usual daily need for it. Nicotinic acid reduces the formation of VLDL-cholesterol in the liver, at the same time reducing the level of free fatty acids (the 'building blocks' of cholesterol) in the circulation.

Nicotinic acid decreases VLDL-cholesterol and LDL-cholesterol levels, while increasing HDL-cholesterol levels by a very substantial 15–25 per cent. It is usually started at doses of around 100–250 mg per day, rising gradually to as much as 4.5–6 g per day. Higher doses may cause liver problems.

The main problem with nicotinic acid is flushing, which can be reduced by taking an aspirin about 15–30 minutes beforehand. Nicotinic acid can add to the effect of blood pressure-lowering drugs, so you should be warned about that if you are asked to take the combination. It can cause gout, a skin condition called acanthosis nigricans, and swelling of the retina in the back of the eye, but happily they all disappear when the drug is stopped. People with active liver disease, diabetes (nicotinic acid can raise blood glucose levels) and gout should probably not take nicotinic acid. If you are taking it you should have a blood test to check your liver and blood glucose every 6 months or so.

It can be given safely with fibrates and bile-acid sequestrants, but not with statins, as it may increase the risk of severe muscle reactions.

Summary

By now you will have realized that the choice of cholesterol-lowering drugs, as with drugs for high blood pressure, is wide, and the drug regimen can be tailored to your particular needs. So your doctors will choose for you a statin, a fibrate, a bile-acid sequestrant or nicotinic acid. The choice depends on your particular pattern of lipids, as well as your total cholesterol level, and also on how well you tolerate the drug you are given. All have their drawbacks, as well as their benefits, so be prepared to have to change them if they are not right for you.

However, drugs alone aren't the answer. To give yourself the best chance of surviving with your kidneys as intact as possible, and of avoiding the heart attack and stroke to which your CKD makes you more vulnerable than others, you have to live the correct lifestyle, too. The next chapters help you to do this.

11

Living well

By now, if you have moderate, stage 3 CKD with an eGFR between 40 and 60, you will have understood that your medical management doesn't entail medicines specifically to treat your kidneys. Instead the main aim is to keep your body in a state that will cause least harm to your kidneys and help to relieve pressures upon them. That's why I have placed so much emphasis so far on blood pressure and cholesterol control. The drugs described in the last two chapters are a mainstay of that programme.

However, they are by no means the only way you can protect your kidneys from further injury. How you live matters a lot, which is why this chapter is about smoking, drinking, eating and exercise. If you follow the rules on these things you will be doing your best to keep your kidneys functioning at least as well as they did at the time of your diagnosis, and you may even improve them.

Smoking

Let's get smoking out of the way first. I have written a little about this stupid, suicidal habit in Chapter 8, so I won't dwell on it, except to state that the combination of carbon monoxide, tars and nicotine does extreme and permanent harm to the delicate kidney structures and mechanisms. You are crazy to smoke if you have CKD. Even one cigarette a day is harmful in that it maintains the narrowing that nicotine causes in the small arteries, including those in the glomeruli, and it presents your kidneys with the job of concentrating cancer-inducing chemicals in the urine. Adding high concentrations of a carcinogen to a kidney already impaired by CKD is, frankly, madness.

So if you smoke, you absolutely *must* stop the habit. How do you go about it?

Stopping smoking

First of all make sure that your aim is to stop, and not just to cut down. Many smokers find, to their surprise, that stopping suddenly is very easy. They take all the cigarettes in their possession and in the house, scrunch them up and throw them in the bin. Then they resolve never to buy any more, and always say 'no', without hesitating, whenever anyone offers them a cigarette. Since the drive to stop smoking in public places, it has become easier than ever to stop. As I'm writing this, the news has just broken that the percentage of smokers in the Scottish population has fallen in the last year by another 1 per cent, continuing the trend for the last 5 years. If these thousands of people can stop, surely you can. After all, you have an extra motivation – the preservation of your kidneys – to help you.

Stopping suddenly raises the bogey of withdrawal symptoms. They vary from agitation, irritation, nervousness and sleeplessness to nothing at all. Doctors like myself who have spent years trying to stop people smoking find that if you have to give up for medical reasons – such as a heart attack or CKD – you hardly ever have withdrawal symptoms, which strongly suggests that they are psychological, rather than physical. In any case, the desire to smoke usually subsides after a week or two, as the feeling of well-being induced by the dropping levels of carbon monoxide, nicotine and tars takes over.

If you still find it difficult to stop, ask your doctor to help you. There are plenty of aids, such as patches, chewing gum and tablets, on offer. But they aren't magical: they will help only if you have the determination to let them. If you have been smoking for years, the best crutch to help you to stop is to change other aspects of your life at the same time. Then you don't associate smoking with your new lifestyle – and that makes it easier to forget cigarettes.

So take plenty of exercise in the first few weeks of stopping: it will help to relieve any tension and also stop you putting on weight as your nicotine-damaged appetite returns. Drink plenty of fluids and eat more fruit – you will find the new tastes (nicotine also damages your sense of taste) exciting and stimulating. Try a new hobby, make new non-smoking friends. And take special care not to succumb to temptation at the time of what was your favourite cigarette of the day.

From the time you stop smoking the break from the habit must be complete: you will never buy or accept another cigarette. Never risk even one cigarette, even at parties where alcohol flows freely and your resistance is low. If you accept one, it is odds-on that you will be smoking as much as ever within weeks.

You owe making the effort to stop smoking to your kidneys, your heart, your lungs and to the future of your family. You will not be on your own. Only one in four people in the UK still smoke. When you stop you will be joining the sensible majority.

Alcohol

There is no such thing as moderate smoking. Every cigarette has the potential to damage your kidneys. Is the same true of alcohol? That is difficult to answer. There is no evidence to link a moderate amount of alcohol with kidney disease. Alcohol tends to open up small arteries, rather than close them, so that some doctors have even argued that it may do 'heart patients', and therefore by inference 'kidney patients', good. However, it all depends on what is meant by 'a little' and on whether the drinker can stick to it. A little can so easily become a lot.

Probably the group of doctors to have done most to clarify the effects of alcohol on health has been the team led by Professor Roger Williams of the Liver Unit at London's King's College Hospital. They drew up the standards for the guidance of doctors.

We were taught that the main organs damaged by alcohol are the brain and the liver, with the heart a close third. Too much alcohol leads to chronic liver disease, dementia and 'alcoholic heart', all of which are lethal. As you have kidney disease, with its predisposition to heart disease and stroke, the precautions doctors would advise you to take if you had heart disease hold for you, too.

First of all there is the general advice about alcohol. We have all had that drummed into us for more than 20 years – ever since the King's College team defined alcohol 'units' and how many units we could drink fairly safely each week before we started to do ourselves damage. That safe level of drinking has finally settled over the years into at most 14 standard units a week for women and 21 for men.

What is a standard drink? When the system started, it was one glass of wine, a half pint of beer, and a single measure of spirits. Since then drinking habits have changed. People have switched from beers to wines, and wine glasses have increased in size from 125 ml or 175 ml to 250 ml. Wine strength has changed, too: 10 years ago its average alcohol content was around 9 per cent. Now it is 12 or 13 per cent. So the single wine glass today contains three of the King's College units. A half bottle of wine has six units, and a bottle 12. It's common for people to drink a half bottle or even a bottle in an evening, and to do this four or five times a week, or even every night. A half bottle of wine five times a week, accepting that you might have two nights off, is 30 units, way above the safe limit for men and women.

Beer strengths have increased, too, with people favouring stronger lagers and beers – often twice the strength of the beers a generation ago – and beer drinkers rarely order half pints now, they drink half litres instead. A half litre is three units. Three of them come to nine units – again much more than you should drink, to be safe, in a day.

Your dilemma, with CKD, is that of every patient with a higher risk of heart attack and stroke. How much can you drink and still not harm yourself? The debate on that subject is fairly fierce in medical circles.

Alcohol tends to open up blood vessels a little: that's why we flush when we drink it. It doesn't increase the tendency of the blood to clot. So in the past many doctors advised people at risk of a heart attack or stroke that they could drink a little every day, because it might do them good.

Unfortunately, that advice may have been wrong. A review, back in the 1990s, by Dr Gareth Beevers, of Birmingham's Dudley Road Hospital (now the City Hospital), established a very strong link between alcohol consumption and high blood pressure. The more his subjects had drunk, the higher were their blood pressures. Dr Beevers proved that alcohol has a direct effect on the heart, even when taken in moderate amounts. Many moderate drinkers had enlarged hearts, high blood pressure and a poor heart reserve in times of crisis. And what was moderate drinking in Dr Beevers' time is very light drinking now.

This is bad news, too, for people with CKD. I don't want to be a killjoy, but if you already have CKD, with an eGFR below 60, we don't know how much extra risk you are taking by drinking more than the odd drink on a few days a week. Having read so far, you will know now that one of your top priorities is to do all you can to keep your blood pressure down. It seems that alcohol won't help you to do that. Since Dr Beevers' report I have changed my attitude to alcohol for all patients at risk of circulation problems. I advise my patients to drink only one or two small drinks in any day and not to drink at all on three or more days a week. In these days of acceptance of alcohol as an accompaniment of almost every meal, that's hard advice to follow, but it makes sense.

Exercise

Just because you have been given the diagnosis of CKD you haven't suddenly become an invalid. There is no reason why you can't become as fit as the next person, and being physically active is crucial to that aim.

You think you are fit enough already? Then try the Harvard Step Test. You can do it at home. All you need is a flight of stairs and a watch. Step from the floor on to the second step (miss the first) of the stairs and down again. Try to do this 30 times a minute for 4 minutes. Time yourself with the watch. You must straighten your knee fully at each step up.

If you get too exhausted to carry on, note down the time that you stopped: it will make a difference to your eventual score. If you have any problems, such as tightness in the chest, stop immediately, rest and tell your doctor about it.

As soon as you finish, sit down quietly and take your pulse for a full 30 seconds starting exactly 1 minute after you stopped. Write down the number of beats immediately, then repeat the 30-second pulse count twice more, starting 2 minutes after you stopped the exercise, then a minute later, writing down the result each time. You can then calculate your recovery index. This is the duration of the exercise in seconds multiplied by 100, divided by double the sum of the three pulse counts.

Take these two examples. Mr A stopped the exercise after 3 minutes 40 seconds (220 seconds) and his 30-second pulse rates were 76, 64 and 60. This gives a score of 22,000 divided by 400, or 55. Miss B completed the 4 minutes and her pulse readings were 66, 57 and 53. She had a score of 24,000 divided by 352, or 68.

Mr A was decidedly unfit. Miss B was fairly fit, but could do better. Try the exercise yourself. If your score is 60 or less you need to be much fitter. You are only 'fair' between 61 and 70, 'good' between 71 and 80, and 'very fit' between 81 and 90. If you score over 90 you are probably already an athlete in training.

Improving your fitness would help your cardiovascular system, and by association your CKD. But you don't have to jog or run to do it. Just walk more, to begin with. If you are a commuter, walk to the station whenever the weather is reasonable, or walk for a bus stop or two before getting on the bus. Use the stairs rather than the lift or escalator. Go by foot to any place within a mile or so, rather than by car. Do, rather than watch, things in your spare time. Go swimming, cycling or walking at weekends. Try gardening or DIY. Any activity is better than none.

Above all do enough exercise to make yourself reasonably out of breath three times a week or more. If you think you might enjoy running, try it, but wear the right footwear if you run on pavements. If an exercise bores you, try something else.

Don't take it too seriously, either. Few people are worse than an exercise bore who constantly talks about his or her times or speeds. Don't buy a stopwatch – competition shouldn't figure high in your leisure time. The idea is to get away from stress, not add to it. A 4-mile walk will get you as fit as if you run the distance in half the time.

Exercise won't kill you. As long as you are sensible about starting, you don't need to consult your doctor beforehand. There are even exercises for people in heart failure, and they feel much the better for them.

Choose your exercise wisely. Don't opt for exercises such as weightlifting: the action of lifting weights or straining muscles while holding your breath is harmful, not beneficial. 'Explosive' sports like squash may also not be right for you. Golf and tennis are more leisurely and probably more acceptable, but if you are new to them take lessons first. Few 'rabbits' last long unless they make rapid progress in their skills.

Daily exercise is all very well, but rest is important, too. You must have your rest periods to let the muscles recover fully. So save 2 days a week for resting. If you are ill, don't try to keep up with your exercise schedule, particularly if you have a virus infection such as the flu or a cold. Never exercise until you are exhausted. Keep it moderate so that you continue to enjoy it. Mixing your activities, too, will help you enjoy the new life more. Take your pick of golf, tennis, cycling, swimming, jogging or simply walking the dog. Do several of them. The variety will give extra interest, and as you see yourself as fitter than most other people it can put your CKD into perspective.

Will the exercise actually improve your chances of long-term survival with CKD? All the studies of people who exercise suggest that it should. People who exercise regularly (and that must include many people who unknowingly have CKD) are less likely to smoke and overeat, tend not to have high blood pressure and have lower blood cholesterol levels than the rest of the population. Their risk of a heart attack is much less than that of couch potatoes.

Exercise also postpones the onset of old age. You get to old age with a straighter back, better neck movements, more mobile joints and more muscle bulk. Older people who are fitter physically feel less depressed and isolated from others. Women who exercise (and men, too) are much less likely to suffer fractures from osteoporosis – a high-risk complication for women with CKD.

Once you start your new life of physical activity, how will you know if you are getting fitter? You will feel better in yourself and be more alert and happier. If you want to prove the benefit beyond doubt, try the Harvard Step Test again after a week of the new you. Your score will have risen dramatically. It will be easier to continue for the full 4 minutes, and your pulse rates will be much slower. Aim for the mid-70 region, and keep around that mark. You don't have to be an Olympic athlete to be fit and well.

12

Food and fluid balance

Knowing what and how much you can eat and drink is essential for anyone with CKD, though the advice changes if you drop from stage 3 (moderate CKD, with an eGFR of 30 to 60) into stage 4 (severe CKD, with an eGFR under 30).

While in stage 3 you still have more than a third of your kidney function left, you are unlikely to have serious symptoms of kidney failure, and your blood tests will not show abnormalities such as anaemia or high potassium and phosphate levels. If you are at this stage you have an excellent chance of remaining at it, and you will have few fluid and food restrictions imposed upon you.

All you need at this stage is a well-balanced and varied eating habit. (I hesitate to call it a diet, since that suggests you are restricted in eating by your illness, and that's the wrong view to take.) So eat a variety of foods, but try to make them as fresh as possible. Many processed foods contain far too much salt, and as we learned in Chapter 2, salt tends to increase your body's fluid volume and blood pressure, both of which are damaging to your kidneys.

So, if you are reading this purely because your GP found by chance that you have an eGFR below 60 but you have no kidney symptoms, then the good news for you is that you can eat virtually what you like – provided it isn't food that is full of salt.

Be wary of salt

Here I must mention Dr Mark MacGregor, Director of our Renal Unit at Crosshouse Hospital in Ayrshire. He has been especially helpful to me in preparing this book, and I'm very grateful to him. When I interviewed him (more about that later) he stressed that in the UK today it is very difficult for people with CKD to find foods that are low enough in salt to protect, rather than worsen, their kidney function.

He told me that the UK government's recommendation for salt intake is less than 5 g (100 mmol) a day – yet even this is too high for CKD patients. You are advised to eat fresh produce rather than processed foods, but it isn't always easy to do so. Salt is everywhere, says Dr MacGregor – in milk, bread, confectionery. He accepts that Marks & Spencer now have a healthy eating guide and label foods with their salt content. Other supermarkets, such as Morrisons and Lidl, have not yet done so, yet their immediate competitors, the Co-op, are doing so. So I unashamedly recommend the Co-op to you. I must admit here to a certain attachment to them, anyway, as my earliest memories include going for the 'messages' (the Scots term for shopping) for my grandmother. I share with Baroness Betty Boothroyd the memory of the family 'divi' number – she apparently did the same for her grandparents.

Sadly for you, take-aways, whether they come from the pizza parlour, the 'Indian' or the chippy, are full of salt, so it's best to cook your own, using ingredients that you know won't push up your salt levels and, with them, your total body fluid volume and blood pressure. As for the big beefburger joints – they should really be off-limits for you.

Food and fluid balance if you are in stage 4 or 5

More restrictions come in if your kidney function has dropped below an eGFR of 30. By then your kidneys aren't dealing with waste products or your electrolyte or fluid balance well enough, and you need extra help. Your first priority is to meet the renal unit dietician, who is expert in dealing with the vagaries of renal failure and its different manifestations in different patients.

She (dieticians are almost always women – I wonder why?) and your renal team (by this time you will be visiting the hospital renal unit regularly) will decide on what your priorities are from the results of your blood tests. The usual problems are higher than normal potassium and phosphate levels, so you will have to reduce or avoid foods rich in these two minerals. Tomatoes, bananas, crisps and coffee are high in potassium, so you may have to do without them. Dairy products such as milk, cheese and eggs are rich in phosphate, so you may have to avoid them, too.

There was a time when people with impending kidney failure were also asked to restrict their protein intake severely, on the grounds that the kidneys could not cope with the management of high levels of protein in the blood. Imagine what was left for people to eat, without various vegetables, dairy products and also meat. You would think there was hardly anything left to eat. Recently the protein restrictions have been less rigid, so that you will be allowed to eat fish and white meat, such as poultry, but to eat red meat only as an occasional treat.

It isn't easy to do without such staple foods at first, but your dietician will help you with advice about various menus that are still tasty and enjoyable. Do, however, stick strictly to her advice, because it can help to postpone the time that you need to go on dialysis, and maybe even help you to avoid it altogether.

By the time you are in stage 4, too, you may be having trouble with your fluid loading. You may be passing less urine than before, and so be tempted to drink more water to compensate. This isn't a good idea. Your dietician and doctor together will plan for you how much fluid you can drink in a day, and the best type of fluids for you. You don't need to measure each drink. You can use the following volumes as a rough, but practical guide:

- standard cup: 180 ml
- full glass or mug: 200 ml
- milk with cereals: 100 ml
- bowl of soup: 150 ml.

Cans and bottles usually have their volumes marked on them.

I don't want to give an average day's intake of fluid for someone in stage 4 or 5 CKD, because it differs between individual patients, and the team treating you will give you the correct advice for you.

Anaemia is another problem that is common in CKD. It may start to appear even when the eGFR is well above 30. If it does, you will probably be given injections of EPO (see Chapter 2) to stimulate your bone marrow into producing more red blood cells. You may be asked to take iron tablets, too. If they upset your stomach (this is less common than it used to be because today's capsules are more stomach-friendly) you can have iron infusions into an arm vein.

Summary

Until now, most of this book has covered what you need to know if you are in stage 3 CKD, with an eGFR between 30 and 60. Your life from now on will combine healthy living with frequent checks on your kidney function, and you will almost certainly be given blood pressure-lowering and cholesterol-lowering treatments. You will be careful about alcohol and salt, and you will avoid tobacco. You can exercise, and most of the time you will feel well. If you can do all that, you almost certainly don't need to worry about your future kidney function. You have a very small chance, only slightly higher than anyone in the general population, of reaching end-stage renal failure, with its consequent need for dialysis and transplant.

The next two chapters describe what to expect if you do reach stages 4 or 5.

13

Dialysis

Here I must again express my thanks to Dr MacGregor. In preparing for this book I was privileged to visit his department, and to watch it working at full strength. It was an eye-opener for me and made me appreciate even more than ever (and I was already a great enthusiast) how good the British NHS is.

If you are one of the small minority of people with CKD whose kidney function continues to deteriorate despite all the care that can be offered, then you have to plan ahead for your time on dialysis or a possible transplant. It is usually fairly easy to predict when that will be. If your kidneys have been worsening over the years, with your eGFR falling and your creatinine levels rising, and symptoms starting to appear, then your nephrologist can construct a chart of the time when you should be joining the dialysis group. You can plan ahead, and visit the dialysis unit in advance, to reduce any fears and apprehensions.

If my visit to the Crosshouse Hospital renal unit is typical, then you have little to fear. I arrived at about midday. There were more than 50 people on the dialysis machines. Some were organizing things for themselves; others needed help from the team of nurses and doctors. So was I looking at a bunch of pale, ill-looking people? Not at all. They all looked healthy and fit. There was a lot of laughter and fun. It was almost like a huge party as patients and nurses chatted and joked together. The place, of course, was spotless, and the laughter and fun didn't detract at all from the professionalism of everyone in the unit, from cleaners and porters to secretaries and nursing and medical staff.

Dr MacGregor, who showed me round, was kind enough to give up his time to spend more than an hour with me. I was staggered to find that there is no 'rationing' in the Ayrshire renal service. Everyone who needs dialysis in the region gets it: old age, for example, is no barrier to receiving it. More than 140 Ayrshire men and women are regular 'haemodialysers' in the Crosshouse unit, with a further 40 or so in the 'satellite' unit in Ayr, 20 miles to the south. And there are more patients who self-dialyse (using peritoneal dialysers) at home. These are big changes from the early days of dialysis, when the upper age limit was 65 and people with diabetes were barred. The alternative then of course was death.

The guidelines on when people with CKD need to begin dialysis are clear. As your kidneys begin to fail completely, you feel unwell. Common symptoms are itch, nausea, vomiting, and the retention of fluid so that your legs swell and you become breathless as your lungs, too, fill with fluid. Anaemia makes this even worse, so that most of the time you feel wretched and tired. Your blood tests confirm the renal failure, with creatinine levels above 500 micromoles/litre – the normal is around 100. The eGFR has dropped, at this stage, below 15 ml/minute.

Dialysis doesn't make your kidneys work better. Sadly, for most people in dialysis, nothing can be done to improve them, and they will continue to deteriorate further until they stop working completely. Instead, dialysis does the work of the kidneys, getting rid of most of the waste that the kidneys would normally excrete, and regulating your fluid and electrolyte balance, so that you lose the excess fluid you have retained since your last 'session', and your sodium, chloride, potassium, phosphate and bicarbonate levels, along with others, are returned to the normal range for people with normal kidneys.

It would be wrong for me to suggest that dialysis holds all the answers for you. It doesn't return you completely to normal, and although many people feel well on it, others are more limited in what they can do, and a minority continue to feel ill. If you are in the last category you may need extra attention to your dialysis regimen, or even to change your type of dialysis, perhaps to 'peritoneal' dialysis.

We use two main types of dialysis – haemodialysis and peritoneal dialysis.

Haemodialysis

The patients I met in the Ayrshire unit were using haemodialysis. That involves placing a 'fistula' (a needle system or a flexible tube) into a vein in an arm, in the neck or just under the collarbone. Blood then flows from you through the fistula into the kidney machine, which removes all that needs to be removed from the blood, which then passes it back into your circulation. The whole process takes around 4 hours, and you do it three times a week.

Although it sounds very limiting to start on dialysis, it actually gives many people more freedom. They feel better, they can get out and about more, eat more varied foods, including more protein, and at the three-times-a-week visit to the unit they make new friends, all of whom understand just what it is like to have CKD. They feel better, lose most of their symptoms – especially the itch and nausea – and they look better, too. Many of the patients in the unit looked fresher than their nurses, who, of course, work very hard during their shifts. (I was there just before a shift ended.)

Of course haemodialysis has its drawbacks. You need to attend a hospital unit to get it. It takes up around 5–7 hours of your time three times a week, depending on the distance from home to hospital. It isn't painful, except that you have local anaesthetic in the arm before the needles are inserted. You have to restrict your fluid intake fairly severely between dialyses, and those dietary restrictions mentioned in the last chapter also apply, but to a lesser extent. You can continue to work, providing you can arrange the times to suit. You may need to organize your dialyses in the evenings, and that can be very tiring after a day's work. Most renal units have shift systems to accommodate people who are still working. It is difficult to take holidays away from your area unless you can organize dialysis in a unit where you will be staying.

Peritoneal dialysis

Peritoneal dialysis (PD) has two forms. One is continuous ambulatory peritoneal dialysis (CAPD); the other is automated peritoneal dialysis (APD). In CAPD you do the dialysis during the day. In APD you are dialysed as you sleep through the night. Their big advantage is that you perform them yourself, at home.

In both types of PD a flexible tube is inserted into your abdomen just below the navel. Its open end lies inside your peritoneum, the fluid-filled cavity that surrounds your stomach and intestines. Your job is to pass specially prepared fluids through the tubing into your peritoneum, and then remove it again. Inside the peritoneum the fluid absorbs the impurities that your kidneys haven't managed to excrete, so that when you remove it, it has acted like a surrogate kidney. You do this four times a day, each time taking around 30–40 minutes.

Here is how it's done:

1 You first wash your hands with a surgical scrub, then wash down the hard surface on which you place the equipment and bags.
2 You take a new bag containing peritoneal dialysis fluid from your box, open it and put it on the cleaned surface. The empty bag that comes along with the full one is placed beside it.
3 You rub your hands again with surgical alcohol, so that they are scrupulously clean before you connect up your bag.
4 Now you join the empty bag to your indwelling catheter – the tube in your abdomen – and place the bag on the floor.
5 You wait for up to 20 minutes to let the old dialysis fluid (that has been inside your abdomen since the last dialysis) drain out into the bag.
6 When the fluid has stopped draining you examine the bag to make sure that it is clear. If it is cloudy it may be infected, and you must tell your doctor at once. You disconnect the old bag and connect the new, full, one.
7 You now hang up your new bag so that it is well above your abdomen, connect it to your catheter line, and let it drain into your abdomen. It will take about 5 minutes.
8 You remove the connection and screw on to the end of your catheter line a 'disconnection cap', which keeps the area clean until the next fluid exchange.
9 You then cut open the bag with the old fluid in it and drain it down the sink, disposing of the empty bag into a medical waste box for incineration.

Sounds complicated? The people I've known who have used PD have quickly adapted to it and have managed to organize their lives around it very well. You are supplied with all the boxes of dialysis bags, dressings and sterilizing fluids, and are properly trained in the techniques before being set free to manage it yourself. It often takes a few months before you are able to look on it as a necessary routine that becomes second nature to you, and during that time you need support, not just for the physical problems you encounter, but also the psychological drawbacks.

It's difficult to come to terms with a permanent tube in your abdominal wall and the need to perform the ritual (for that is what it becomes) four times a day. Your body image can suffer, because you have a swollen abdomen most of the time. But if you can manage it well it gives you a personal freedom that is more difficult to achieve if you have to visit your own hospital three times a week.

The main complication of either type of peritoneal dialysis is peritonitis. If you are not absolutely scrupulous about infection control and prevention, you can get an infection, peritonitis, through the catheter. This produces fever, nausea and vomiting, and abdominal cramps and aches, and it can even be life-threatening. Bouts of peritonitis can leave scarring inside the abdomen that makes future CAPD impossible, so that you have to revert to haemodialysis. You are therefore trained in the techniques to avoid peritonitis at all costs.

The advantages of CAPD are that you can do it at home, and it is easy to arrange for all the paraphernalia to be delivered to you on holiday. Indira, our patient described earlier, in Chapter 4, was easily able to organize her CAPD materials when she went regularly to Cyprus on holiday. Inside the EU, dialysis is provided free for anyone on holiday, and most of the rest of the world has kidney failure services that will help you. However, before you plan your holiday check up on how safe they are. In some countries some dialysis units are not free from hepatitis viruses, and you must not risk going to them.

An added thought: if you are considering travelling abroad, make sure that you mention your kidney problem to your insurers. If you haven't done so, and you become ill or are involved in an accident, you may not have insurance cover for any kidney complications, and that can cripple you financially.

Note, too, that although the EU system provides for emergency medical care, it is not necessarily free, and doesn't cover very high expenses such as the cost of an ambulance to get you home. If you are planning a holiday in the EU, you still have to take this into account when insuring against emergencies. Information about the European Health Insurance Card (EHIC, the replacement of the old E111) is available in post offices and will point you in the right direction.

CAPD can give you some abdominal pain and swelling, but most people manage to come to terms with them. You can go to work with CAPD, provided that you can arrange to do the dialysis, say, in your lunch break. Diet and fluid restrictions are not quite as strict as those for people on haemodialysis.

Body image and sex life on dialysis

Once you are on dialysis, of either type, you will feel and look much better. However, you have to come to terms with the fact that you may look different. On haemodialysis the fistula will be noticeable, and may even 'buzz' a little. On PD your stomach will bulge a little, and there is a catheter sticking out from the front of it. Nevertheless it shouldn't stop you enjoying the sex life you had before. So do feel free to discuss this and all its implications with your partner and doctors. It's a good idea for your partner to be brought into all the planning well beforehand so that nothing comes as a shock.

Some men with CKD find they have difficulties in producing and maintaining an erection. Part of this may be their psychological reaction to their new body image, and it can be treated with good advice from the renal team. Part of it may be physical, and it can be managed with drugs such as sildenafil (Viagra). The National Kidney Federation has a brilliant website at <www.kidney.org.uk>, which deals in detail with ways to overcome sexual difficulties. Anaemia may be one cause of sexual problems in men and women, and its treatment (with EPO and iron) can help to minimize them.

Having children

CKD lowers the sperm count in men and makes women less fertile. If you have CKD and want children, it has to be said that you have difficulties to face. A low sperm count does not always prevent men from becoming fathers, even when they are in stage 4 or 5, but it is less likely. By the time women reach the stage of dialysis they are usually no longer ovulating, making pregnancy highly unlikely. However, if you are still having periods there is always a chance that you will conceive. If you don't want children then it is best to use contraception.

Pregnancy in women in stages 1 to 3 usually proceeds normally, but if you become pregnant in stage 4 or 5, when you are already on dialysis, you face considerable difficulties in bringing the pregnancy to full term and having a normally healthy baby. If you want to conceive in this stage of CKD you should first talk your plans over with your doctors. In the mean time you should always use contraception until you are sure that this is the right thing for you.

Interestingly, having a baby after you have had a kidney transplant is less difficult, and usually has a better outcome, than if you are on dialysis. Even so, you should still discuss it with your doctors before making the decision.

14

Kidney transplants

Dialysis is only second best as a treatment for end-stage kidney failure. A successful kidney transplant gives you a much better quality of life, as long as it is free of complications.

Harry had his transplant as long ago as 1983, when he was 45, a year after he suddenly developed acute kidney failure. The initial cause of his sudden kidney collapse was never found, but it soon became clear that it was irreversible, and he was treated with haemodialysis. Happily he only had to wait for a year for his kidney, and it worked extremely well. This year he celebrates his quarter century with his new kidney. He is planning a holiday in New Zealand to visit family there, and his doctors don't foresee any problems.

His current eGFR is only 25 ml/minute and his serum creatinine is 220 micromoles/litre, well above the normal of around 100. However these two measures of kidney function, which put him firmly into stage 4, have been stable at around this level for the past 5 years. He has no symptoms, feels well and is determined to enjoy life. He has taken out full insurance for his trip to New Zealand and his insurers know his 'kidney history'. He is now 69; he worked until the state retirement age of 65, and he considers himself very lucky to have been given a second chance at life 25 years ago.

Harry was given his kidney from a young man who had died in a road accident. Like all the other kidney recipients I have met, he talks enthusiastically of the feeling of well-being that the new organ gave him. He felt almost instantly better physically and mentally, and is so grateful to the family of the donor for consenting to the transplant.

Harry's story is fairly typical. The new kidney doesn't often work quite as well as a completely healthy kidney, but it usually works well enough to make you feel human again. There are drawbacks. You must take drugs to stop you rejecting the donated organ, but over the last few years anti-rejection management has become very skilled, so that far fewer transplanted kidneys have to be removed. Today 95 per cent of all transplanted kidneys still work well after a year, and half of them are still working well after 15 years. Many, of course, like Harry's and Peter Leslie's (I wrote about him in Chapter 2: his transplant has lasted 43 years to date) last much longer than 15 years, and as transplant surgery progresses we expect the average duration of transplanted kidneys to extend by many more years. The transplants of today should last much longer than those of 20 years ago.

Kidney donation

The most effective transplants are from living donors who have agreed to give a kidney to a relative or a friend. If you wish to do this, you must be healthy and have no history of serious illness that might have affected the kidneys. You will be guided by a transplant co-ordinator working closely with the kidney team, and you will be fully informed about your risks. No one will put pressure on you, and of course you will not be paid for the donation. In the UK, and in all modern countries with good renal services, it is illegal to buy a kidney from someone or to pay someone to donate a kidney. However, because you will be undergoing surgery and have several weeks off work, you should get compensation for any loss of earnings.

Giving a kidney carries the same small risk that any operation under anaesthetic has: today this risk is tiny. It takes a few months to return to your old fitness level, but that is a minor drawback to set against seeing the huge improvement your kidney has made in the recipient's life. In the long run, your remaining kidney increases its work to compensate for the loss, and you will not notice any difference in your own health.

The biggest problem about kidney transplants is not medical – it is that we can't get enough donors.

I'm writing this chapter in January 2008, when the great political news is that the British Prime Minister, Gordon Brown, has swung his political weight behind a new approach to organ donation. He wants to bring into the UK a system of 'opting out', rather than 'opting in' for donations. Simply put, that means that it is assumed that organs can be taken for transplant from a person who has died suddenly in hospital provided that he or she has not expressly forbidden this in life – in effect opting out of the transplant system.

Our present system, of 'opting in', involves people carrying donor cards with them wherever they are, so that the transplant team have hard evidence that they were willing to be donors. This system has led to the UK having one of the lowest organ donation rates in Europe, with just 13 donors per million population. Only a quarter of the population carry donor cards, and only a fraction of this quarter, of course, is ever in the tragic situation of becoming a donor. And although 90 per cent of people say that they support organ donation, only 35 per cent of them actually agree when they have to make the decision suddenly in a family tragedy.

The result of the 'opting in' policy is that we now have 8,000 people in Britain waiting for an organ transplant (mostly waiting for a kidney), around 1,000 of whom will die before they receive their organ. Something drastic must be done to redress this, despite the fears of some people that changing to an 'opting out' system might lead to body parts being removed against people's wishes.

There is now a UK Organ Donation Task Force, which has the prime aim of increasing organ donations. The idea is to create a UK-wide network of organ-retrieval teams and to expand the work of donor transplant co-ordinators. NHS staff will be trained to look upon organ donation as normal, rather than unusual. The Task Force is hoping to bring about a rise in donors of about 50 per cent in the next 5 years, aside from the switch to 'opting out'. This should save about 1,000 lives a year in the UK.

To illustrate the need for this change in policy, on 17 January 2008, *The Herald* (one of the two national papers in Scotland) highlighted the story of Katherine Blenman. She, her mother, her sister and her brother have all had kidney transplants because of their inherited polycystic kidneys. Her transplant has, she says, 'revolutionized her life'. Her two daughters may also need new kidneys one day. 'I don't think people realize', she continues, 'how important it is to join the register [of donors]. Anything that leads to more people signing up is a good thing.'

Hear, hear!

There are plenty of people and organizations that will support Katherine and her family. The final section in this book lists the organizations to whom people with CKD can turn for help. They are all excellent and I recommend them to you.

Useful addresses

Patients' associations

There is a wealth of organizations to which you can turn to learn more about CKD, and they are a huge source of strength and reassurance when you are in need. Among them are three or four patients' associations:

British Kidney Patient Association (BKPA)
Bordon
Hants GU35 9JZ
Tel.: 01420 472021/2
Website: www.britishkidney-pa.co.uk

Kidney Research UK
King's Chambers
Priestgate
Peterborough PE1 1FG
Tel.: 0845 070 7601
Helpline: 0845 300 1499
Website: www.kidneyresearchuk.org

National Kidney Federation (NKF)
The Point
Coach Road
Shireoaks
Worksop
Nottinghamshire S81 8BW
Tel.: 01909 544999
Helpline: 0845 601 0209
Website: www.kidney.org.uk

If you have diabetes as well as CKD, please contact:

Diabetes UK
10 Parkway
London NW1 7AA
Tel.: 020 7424 1000
Helpline: 0845 120 2960
Website: www.diabetes.org.uk

Internet sites

There are also internet sites from which you can glean practically all the information you need about every aspect of CKD. I include a few that my friends in the renal service recommend.

http://body.orpheusweb.co.uk
This website covers the work of the British Organ and Donation Society (BODY), which gives information on transplants and donation. While their own former site (www.argonet.co.uk/body) is being rebuilt, you might prefer to contact them at BODY, Balsham, Cambridge CB21 4DL; tel.: 01223 893636.

www.dh.gov.uk/en/Healthcare/Healthadvicefortravellers/index.htm
This website answers questions on health topics, immunizations and precautions to take before travelling abroad. Information about the European Health Insurance Card (EHIC, the replacement of the old E111) is available from this website.

www.eurodial.org
This website is run by the International Dialysis Organisation, for the care of people travelling throughout Europe.

www.globaldialysis.com
Use this website for holiday and travel information for dialysis patients worldwide.

www.kidney.org.uk/Medical-Info/drugs/vacc2.html
This is part of the NKF website and informs you about the medicines and vaccinations you can and can't have if you have had a kidney transplant.

www.nephron.com
This website is devoted to the details of kidney diseases.

www.patients-association.com
This is the website of the Patients Association, which advises you on your rights as a patient.

www.renalinfo.com
This website gives ideas on how to plan your future treatment.

http://renux.dmed.ed.ac.uk/EdRen
This is the link to the website <www.edren.org> which is the site of the Edinburgh Renal Unit: useful for wide-ranging information about CKD.

www.uktransplant.org.uk
This is an NHS website informing you about organ transplants and organ donation.

Index